Handbook of Service User Involvement
in Nursing and Healthcare Research

In memory of Ursula Hawgood, who worked with us,
inspired us and involved us.

Handbook of Service User Involvement in Nursing and Healthcare Research

Elizabeth Morrow
Research Fellow
National Nursing Research Unit
King's College London

Annette Boaz
Lecturer in Translational Research
Division of Health and Social Care Research
King's College London

Sally Brearley
Honorary Senior Research Fellow in Public
and Patient Involvement
National Nursing Research Unit
King's College London

Fiona Ross
Dean and Professor of Primary Care Nursing
Faculty of Health and Social Care Sciences
St George's, University of London

WILEY-BLACKWELL

A John Wiley & Sons, Ltd., Publication

This edition first published 2012 © 2012 by Elizabeth Morrow, Annette Boaz, Sally Brearley and Fiona Ross
Wiley-Blackwell is an imprint of John Wiley & Sons, formed by the merger of Wiley's global Scientific, Technical and Medical business with Blackwell Publishing.

Registered Office
John Wiley & Sons, Ltd, The Atrium, Southern Gate, Chichester, West Sussex, PO19 8SQ, UK

Editorial Offices
9600 Garsington Road, Oxford, OX4 2DQ, UK
The Atrium, Southern Gate, Chichester, West Sussex, PO19 8SQ, UK
111 River Street, Hoboken, NJ 07030-5774, USA

For details of our global editorial offices, for customer services and for information about how to apply for permission to reuse the copyright material in this book please see our website at www.wiley.com/wiley-blackwell.

Library of Congress Cataloging-in-Publication Data

Handbook of service user involvement in nursing and healthcare research/Elizabeth Morrow ... [et al.].
    p.; cm.
  Includes bibliographical references and index.
  ISBN-13: 978-1-4443-3472-2 (pbk. : alk. paper)
  ISBN-10: 1-4443-3472-7 (pbk. : alk. paper)
1. Nursing–Research. 2. Medical care–Research. 3. Medical personnel and patient.
I. Morrow, Elizabeth, 1975–
  [DNLM: 1. Nursing Research. 2. Health Services Research. 3. Patient Participation.
4. Professional-Patient Relations. WY 20.5]
  RT81.5.H36 2012
  610.73072–dc23

                             2011015202

A catalogue record for this book is available from the British Library.

This book is published in the following electronic formats: ePDF 9781444347029; Wiley Online Library 9781444347050; ePub 9781444347036; Mobi 9781444347043

Set in 10/12.5pt Times by SPi Publisher Services, Pondicherry, India
Printed and bound in Malaysia by Vivar Printing Sdn Bhd

1   2012

Contents

Contributors

The following people have kindly worked with us in the preparation of this book to share some of their experiences of service user involvement in research:

- *Sophie Auckland*, User Involvement Manager for Guy's and St Thomas' Foundation Trust and King's College London Biomedical Research Centre explains her experiences of informing and advising academic and clinical research staff in a wide range of research areas including laboratory research, clinical trials and qualitative studies.
- *Sheila Donovan*, Research Fellow at the Faculty of Health and Social Care Sciences, Kingston University and St George's University of London, explains some of the issues that can arise in relation to older service users' views about payment.
- *Jennifer Laws*, a Researcher and Teaching Fellow at Durham University, provides an insight into managing diverse expectations whilst working with mental health service users to develop peer-support and advocacy services.
- *Professor Colin Torrance*, *Dr Keith Weeks* and *Christine Wilson* explain their views about embedding service user involvement in learning organisations. They are part of a research team at the University of Glamorgan, investigating the use of clinical simulation and virtual learning environments to educate healthcare professionals.
- *Hazel Thornton*, an Independent Advocate for Quality in Research and Healthcare, provides insights into service user involvement in clinical trials for breast cancer treatment.
- *Sally Crowe*, a consultant in Patient and Public Involvement, draws on her experiences of the practical and emotional aspects of involvement to provide advice about hearing the voices of those who are very sick.
- *Dr Patricia Grocott*, Reader Palliative Wound Care, King's College London, and *Elizabeth Pillay*, Nurse Consultant, St Thomas' Hospital London, explain how they are working in partnership with the charity DebRA UK to involve people with chronic and severe skin conditions in research.
- *Jennifer Newman*, Consumer Liaison Officer for the National Institute for Health Research Medicines for Children Research Network, explains her experiences of working to involve parents, carers, children and young people in the networks' activities.
- *Professor Jane Coad*, based at Coventry University, explains some of her experiences of involving children and young people in the development of health services using participatory arts-based methods.
- *Amy Feltham* from YoungMinds provides a young person's view of VIK (Very Important Kid) panel and explains how getting the little things right helps make sure the big things run smoothly.

- *Julie Wray*, Researcher/Healthcare Professional/Survivor, explains her views on embracing the patient/carer voice and the importance of caring for the person not the illness.
- *Christine Wilson* explains how she has developed interactive methods – a Living Library – to help engage healthcare professionals and researchers in dialogue with people with mental health problems.
- *The Sunderland family* from Northumberland provide an insight into the research they did with their father before his death to mesothelioma in 2009.
- *Nazira Visram*, an experienced patient representative and Macmillan Trainer, discusses ideas for moving forward and sustaining collective service user efforts alongside contributing to experiential learning and self-management programmes for cancer care.
- *Rory Byrne*, based at the University of Manchester, gives a user-researcher's perspective of mental health service user involvement.
- *Professor Jane Coad* describes a collaborative project with the children's charity CLIC Sargent and some of the lessons learnt about how to evaluate young people's experiences of involvement.
- *Antje Lindenmeyer*, Senior Research Fellow, Warwick Diabetes Care Research and Education User Group, explains her experiences of assessing the benefits of service user involvement with lay people who have an active interest in the experiences and care of people living with diabetes.

About the authors

Dr Elizabeth Morrow   I started working in healthcare research in 1999 when I took up a Research Assistant post at the Faculty of Health and Social Care Sciences based at St George's Hospital and jointly run by Kingston University. Before that I trained as a geologist and had briefly worked for the National Trust showing visitors around Cornish engine houses. In my new career, working under the direction of Professor Fiona Ross, I began to learn about research with people, the health system and something about professional cultures. Over the years I have worked on nursing research studies and service development projects and have enjoyed building relationships with a wide range of service users and their representative organisations. In 2003, I was lead researcher on the National Institute for Health Research Service Delivery and Organisation PIN project (Patient and public involvement in nursing, midwifery and health visiting research), led by Professor Ross. My doctoral thesis went on to look at the development of service user involvement in health research in the United Kingdom and Australia. My thesis argued that current knowledge and conceptualisations of service user involvement in health research tend to underplay the significance of external influencing factors such as established notions of what constitutes health research. The research I undertook showed that although tensions about professional power over service user involvement in health research cannot be escaped, they can be better understood by examining the reasons behind resistance and discomfort. These reasons may be entirely valid, but where there is uncertainty there is also the potential to develop new knowledge through language development, new epistemological stances, and subjective experiences and views. I now work as a Research Fellow for the National Nursing Research Unit based at King's College London. My research interests include exploring the contribution that service users can, and should, make to contemporary healthcare policy and practice. With Annette Boaz, Sally Brearley and other colleagues I teach service user involvement in research at King's College London.

Dr Annette Boaz   I have an ongoing interest in the roles patients, carers and the public play in research and I am currently a Lecturer in Translational Research at King's College London. I am leading a project exploring the relationship between public and patient involvement in research and public engagement in science. I am also supporting biomedical researchers with an interest in service user involvement in their research. I have previously worked at the universities of Oxford and Warwick, carrying out research in a wide variety of policy areas, completing evaluations for the UK Cabinet Office and Home Office. I also worked briefly in the Policy Research Programme at the UK

Department of Health. At Warwick, I was involved in the evaluation of the Better Government for Older People action research programme, working alongside a group of older people committed to improving services for an ageing population.

Sally Brearley   I trained and worked as a physiotherapist in Manchester in the 1970s. In the mid-1980s, I gained a BSc in Nursing Studies at King's College London. For my final year's dissertation I reviewed research on what was then called patient participation. During my time at King's College London, Fiona Ross was a lecturer there. After an MA in Social Anthropology, and whilst my children were small, I became interested in patient stories and got involved in a number of patient organisations. Meeting up again with Fiona Ross and with Elizabeth Morrow, both then at the Faculty of Health and Social Care Sciences Kingston University and St George's University of London, we began our collaboration on service user involvement in research, which has now spanned more than a decade. Currently I am an honorary fellow at the Faculty of Health and Social Care Sciences Kingston University and St George's University of London, and at the National Nursing Research Unit, King's College London. I am still active in a number of organisations representing patients and the public, and in supporting the National Health Service.

Prof Fiona Ross   I did my first degree at Edinburgh University, where I trained to be a nurse. After qualification I worked as a district nurse in London where I enjoyed the privilege of looking after people in their own homes, where they could choose how and in what way they received their care. Perhaps it was these beginnings that led me to a PhD that focused on patient-held information, in relation to medication management. Later research opportunities built my interest in how to better work with patients in the co-production of research. I believe research should not be the preserve of the professional, but should be done with, and on account of, the people, patients and their families, whom it should ultimately benefit. This book is the outcome of some of that thinking, produced by a talented and collaborative group of researchers, whom I have been privileged to work with. Along the way I have done a number of jobs and held Chairs in Primary Care Nursing, been the Director of the National Nursing Research Unit at King's College London, and I am currently the Dean of a large Faculty of Health and Social Care Sciences, run as a joint venture by Kingston University and St George's, University of London.

Preface

In nursing and healthcare practice, there is a long history of working with patients to understand their health needs and to assess the best options for treatment and care. Nurses and other healthcare practitioners – including midwives, health visitors, occupational health workers, community health workers, or another person trained and knowledgeable in nursing or other allied health professions or public/community health – have tended to make the most of this close relationship with the patient, to try to see things from the patient's perspective.

As we see it, nursing and healthcare research is about the generation of knowledge to inform practice, education, management and policy development that relates to these professional roles. It can be undertaken by paid and unpaid researchers from many different clinical and non-clinical backgrounds, as well as in education, management, policy development and student research projects. In recent years, across many countries, there have been widespread changes in research policy and practice which aim to involve 'service users' (patients, carers and the public) more directly and actively in all aspects of health and social care research. In health policy and research literatures the term 'service user' is generally used to mean patients, carers and members of the public; however, alternative terms such as 'patient', 'public', 'consumer', 'citizen', 'lay representative' and 'user representative' are also in use. However, the language of involvement is continuously developing and is contested.

This book looks at service user involvement at a time when political and professional support is growing rapidly as part of a trend towards improving public engagement in governance of public institutions. Changes are being seen to involve the public in the organisation and delivery of healthcare services, the education of healthcare professionals, and in all aspects of health and social care research. These changes place new emphasis on gaining a balance between developing valid generalisable knowledge and benefiting the community that is being researched.

Recent politically driven forms of involvement are distinctly different from longerstanding emancipatory movements where people who are directly affected by the issues seek to bring about change. Growing numbers of service users are embarking on their own personal health research, as well as 'user-led', 'user-controlled' and 'survivor' research. Research commissioners are also more open to funding user-led research and the leadership role of service users is beginning to be recognised.

Increasingly, demonstrating a commitment to working with service users is a condition of being awarded research funding, but it is also becoming a sign of quality in research. There is some evidence that involving service users at different stages of the research process can help to improve research studies in terms of the questions they seek to address, how they are carried out and the impact of the findings. There is stronger evidence that service user involvement has an impact on the service users and researchers who are involved in the process.

At the outset, the realities of involving service users in research can be daunting for new and experienced researchers. Service users may also be apprehensive or have uncertainties about what the process will entail. Nurses and other healthcare professionals often need to combine their research role with their clinical roles and this duality is a potential cause of ambiguity and tension when inviting service users to work alongside them as partners. Knowing who to involve and how to involve different people requires sensitivity and understanding, as well as an appreciation of how research can be perceived as being remote from the 'real world'. Researchers need to be aware of processes of negotiation, mutuality and respect in their work with service users. There are specific types of ethical and legal issues that differ from involving people as subjects in research. There are research governance, management and resource issues that mean that researchers need to be able to plan and record service user involvement activities. Researchers can make use of models of service user involvement and techniques to enable service users' ideas to be brought forward and made use of in research.

This book is an introduction to service user involvement in research which will be useful for anyone working in, or learning about, nursing or healthcare research. We have purposely used the term 'research teams' in the book to convey the fact that researchers do not work in isolation, and, that the ideal situation is for researchers and service users to learn about service user involvement in research together.

The book provides some insight into service users' diverse expectations about involvement, the types of contributions they might make, and the impact their involvement is likely to have. The key ideas and tools included through the book could be useful for established healthcare researchers to support service user involvement in research design, writing proposals for research funding and working to embed learning across research organisations. It focuses on service user involvement in UK and European contexts but readers from other countries are likely to recognise the issues and be able to make use of many of the ideas that are put forward.

The idea for the book came from a series of studies and collaborations between the authors. In 2003, three of the authors were involved in a scoping study commissioned by the National Co-ordinating Centre for Service Delivery and Organisation Research and Development Nursing and Midwifery Subgroup (Ross et al. 2004). The overall aim of the scoping study was to identify priorities for research funding in nursing and midwifery in England by reviewing the literature, consulting professionals and stakeholders, and conducting discussions with consumer representatives. Involvement of members of 38 Community Health Councils during the scoping exercise had a significant influence on the depth of information we gained and proved to us that involvement was achievable and that it added value to research (Smith et al. 2005). In 2004, we were commissioned to undertake the National Institute for Health Research Service Delivery and Organisation PIN project (Patient and public involvement in nursing, midwifery and health visiting research). This study again involved service users, but more actively in the review process itself. Between us, our collective experiences gave us confidence to aim for more substantial service user involvement as part of a collaborative multi-method approach (Smith et al. 2008).

Through these and other studies, we have learnt about the practical aspects of service user involvement, such as the need to meet people on their own terms, how to build relationships through personalised communication and understanding that every service user has a unique contribution to make. Working with service users helped us to overcome some of our own apprehensions about involvement and to find better ways to work in partnership. Of course, we have also been informed, influenced and inspired by the work of other researchers and service users, and what is written in the research literature. We have taken this learning forward in our own work and contributed to developing guidelines on service user involvement for nurse researchers (Royal College of Nursing 2007).

Our intention for this book is to share some of this learning in a useful handbook. We would not wish for it to be seen as a set of instructions. We see it as a collection of ideas and tools to help inform the design and undertaking of service user involvement in nursing and healthcare research. It is a resource for anyone who wants to find out more or to make connections with individuals and organisations who are leading the way in developing service user involvement. Through the book, you will find case studies written by service users and researchers, and from further afield in health and social care. These contributions help to bring the topic of service user involvement in research to life and to highlight key issues from the perspectives of those who have experienced service user involvement.

References

Ross, F., Smith, E., Mackenzie, A., and Masterson, A. (2004) Identifying research priorities in nursing and midwifery service delivery and organisation: a scoping study. *International Journal of Nursing Studies*, 41 (5): 547–58.

Royal College of Nursing (2007) *User Involvement in Research: Guidelines for Nurse Researchers.* London, U.K.: Royal College of Nursing. (Available from: http://www.rcn.org.uk/)

Smith, E., Ross, F., Mackenzie, A., and Masterson, A. (2005) Developing a service user framework to shape priorities for nursing and midwifery research. *Journal of Research in Nursing*, 1 (10): 107–18.

Smith, E., Ross, F., Donovan, S., Manthorpe, G., Brearley, S., Sitzia, J., and Beresford, P. (2008) Service user involvement in the design and undertaking of nursing, midwifery and health visiting research. *International Journal of Nursing Studies*, 45: 298–315.

Structure of the book

We have divided the book into three main parts: Part I (Preparing), Part II (Learning) and Part III (Evaluating). Each chapter begins with a summary of key issues covered in the chapter and ends with key principles for practice. We have used figures and summary boxes throughout to make the material accessible for reference purposes and for teaching and learning.

Part I   Preparing

Part I begins by introducing the concept of service user involvement in nursing and healthcare research and explaining some of the different ways of approaching the topic. It then sets out some of the political and research contexts of involvement and moves to engage the public more actively in a wide range of professional areas of working. We then look at some of the underlying drivers for service user involvement and the perspectives different stakeholders might have of the issues. We outline what is currently known about impact and some of the challenges associated with building knowledge to inform research practice, such as focusing research efforts and sharing existing learning. Chapter 2 concerns concepts of involvement, including the concepts of 'service users', 'involvement', 'representation', 'experiential knowledge', 'empowerment' and 'participation'. We look at the models that authors have devised to help explain the types of relationships that can exist between service users and researchers in research. These include a ladder of participation, levels of involvement (consultation, collaboration, control) and a continuum of participation. We present our own broad theoretical framework for approaching service user involvement at the end of Chapter 2. It sets out four interrelated components for personal and professional learning: context, methods, roles and outcomes. Chapter 3 moves on to discuss how to design involvement, including practical advice about deciding who to involve; building in opportunities and time for involvement, costing and payments; and research ethics and governance issues to be aware of. The final chapter of the part (Chapter 4) presents ideas for establishing good working relationships including making connections with service users, developing working environments, being clear about roles and responsibilities, explaining legal and ethical issues, providing training and support, effective communication, and opportunities for feedback and reflection. We look at some of the issues associated with embedding service user involvement in research organisations, how organisations can spread learning, build expertise and develop best practice for ways of working and support systems.

Part II   Learning

Part II focuses on involving and learning from different types of service users. It begins by looking at issues of involving patients and clients who are receiving health care, and people who are very sick or have rare clinical conditions (Chapter 5). Involvement over the life course is an important issue and some of the more specific issues of involving children, young people, adults and older people are outlined in Chapter 6. Chapter 7 discusses the multiple barriers and circumstances that affect seldom-heard groups including lack of awareness, communication barriers and access issues. It sets out some key issues in relation to involving people with physical disabilities, the deaf and people who are hard of hearing, people who are blind or partially sighted, people with learning disabilities, people with degenerative cognitive impairment, people with mental health problems, and Black and minority ethnic groups. Chapter 8 focuses on service user-led research. It explains how individual service users, sometimes with the support of their family members or carers, may undertake their own research to better understand an illness or the options for treatment or care. We then look at the types of research work that volunteer networks, service user-led organisations, charities and not-for-profit organisations might undertake or be involved in, and the emerging roles of experienced service user representatives and academic service user researchers.

Part III   Evaluating

Part III focuses broadly on issues of evaluating service user involvement. Chapter 9 begins by looking at known indicators of success which research teams can use to plan and assess whether they are meeting established ideas of good practice. The chapter then explains why it is important to document service user involvement work as part of recording research processes and demonstrating active and direct participation of service users. Research teams can also make use of a range of reflective techniques to examine issues about the quality of involvement processes, for example reflective diaries, feedback and evaluation forms, and reflective interviewing. By using reflexivity and considering quality at an organisational and research systems level, research teams may also be able to contribute towards more supportive research environments and to challenge any barriers to involvement. Chapter 10 focuses on issues of impact, including suggestions on how to recognise impact, record impact and report impact. Understanding impact is important because it can help to show whether involvement is effective and to demonstrate the benefits and drawbacks in different research contexts. Chapter 11 takes a different look at the issues by examining international developments in service user involvement in research across Europe, USA, Canada, Australia and New Zealand, and in developing countries. Different countries tend to favour different types of concepts which may be related to service user involvement, for example patient-centred care, consumer engagement, patient participation, or patient and public involvement. The chapter provides details of government-funded and non-government-funded organisations which provide information, funding and support for service user involvement activities internationally.

Chapter 12 brings a close to the book by presenting summary conclusions and looking at some of the wider implications of service user involvement for enhancing evidence-based practice and enriching healthcare professional education. For those readers who are also teachers, the chapters of this book could be used as an outline curriculum for a session or module on service user involvement in nursing or healthcare research. Example topics for student discussions, group work and essay questions are provided. The final sections of the chapter look at the issues of service user involvement in relation to developing professional roles and securing service users' commitment to involvement.

Acknowledgements

This book was informed and inspired by the aforementioned contributors and many other researchers and service users who we have had the pleasure of working with. We would like to personally acknowledge the following people: Dr Patricia Grocott, Reader at the Florence Nightingale School of Nursing and Midwifery, King's College London, and Professor Margaret O'Connor at the School of Nursing and Midwifery, Monash University, for their support and advice on work which led to this book. Dr Janette Bennett provided advice on concepts of knowledge and power.

We would like to thank colleagues who have worked with us on various service user involvement projects, in particular: Professor Peter Beresford at the Centre of Citizen Participation Brunel University; John Sitzia, R&D Director at Worthing and Southlands Hospitals; Dr Felicity Callard, Service User Research Enterprise Institute of Psychiatry, King's College London; Professor Jill Manthorpe, Social Care Workforce Research Unit; and Dr Christopher McKevitt, Nina Fudge, Sophie Auckland and Dr Josephine Ocloo at King's College London. Thanks to Sarah Buckland and Helen Hayes, INVOLVE Support Unit.

Thank you to the many service users who have given their time and inspired us in various ways. In particular, we would like to acknowledge the contribution of members of the service user reference group who worked with us on the National Institute for Health Research Service Delivery and Organisation PIN project (Patient and public involvement in nursing, midwifery and health visiting research). Thanks to them and their organisations: Age Concern; AIMS (Association for Improvements in the Maternity Services); BLISS – The premature baby charity; British Council for Disabled People; British Heart Foundation; Cancer Research UK; Carers London/UK; Clifford Beers Foundation; Diabetes UK; Redbridge Primary Care Trust; Voluntary Groups Advisory Council Diabetes UK; Friends of the Elderly; Folk.US; London Voices & Croydon Voices; National Children's Bureau; National Childbirth Trust; Northumberland User Voice; Patient and Public Involvement Forum Royal College of General Practitioners; Quality Research in Dementia; Shaping our Lives; and Values into Action. Guest advisors to the group were Mr Tim Twelvetree, Institute for Public Health Research and Policy, and Ms Jayne Pyper, Ovacome.

Part I

Preparing

Chapter 1

Perspectives and expectations

Key summary points

- *Approaching service user involvement*: Service user involvement in research means different things to different people, however, the term is generally used to mean the active and direct participation of service users in the commissioning, design, undertaking or evaluation of research. Approaching service user involvement requires asking questions including: Why should researchers involve service users? What are the purposes and the benefits? How can the process be successful and productive? Who should be involved to ensure representation and diversity? When should service users be involved and at which stages of the research?
- *Political and research contexts of involvement*: Across many Westernised nations there is strong interest in engaging the public more actively in a wide-range of professional areas of working, including healthcare delivery, service design and health and social care research. Diversity is an important concept in relation to both the contexts of service user involvement and to the professionals and service users it concerns. At the same time many of the challenges and opportunities of service user involvement are shared between professional groups and across disciplinary boundaries.
- *Historical roots and social movements*: It is important to appreciate that moves to involve service users in a wide-range of professional activities have come about because of the culmination of a series of historical events, rather than a one-off policy directive. The drivers for service user involvement include historical and ethical reasons such as challenges to medical authority, changing roles of patients in policy, user-led research, democratisation of public services and public response to professional scandals.
- *Perspectives of service user involvement*: In general, research funders are looking for a commitment to service user involvement including making sure it is appropriate to the research and that there is adequate planning and budgeting. Researchers may hope that involving service users will help them to secure funding and to improve the quality and outcomes of the research they undertake. Service users have a wide range of personal motives for wanting to be involved in research. As a minimum they should be given sufficient information about their involvement in the research, to be respected, to be involved in ways that suit them, and to be acknowledged for their contributions to the research.

Handbook of Service User Involvement in Nursing and Healthcare Research, First Edition.
Elizabeth Morrow, Annette Boaz, Sally Brearley and Fiona Ross.
© 2012 Elizabeth Morrow, Annette Boaz, Sally Brearley and Fiona Ross.
Published 2012 by Blackwell Publishing Ltd.

- *What is known about the impact of involvement*: There are numerous strong accounts to suggest that the quality and outcomes of research studies can be improved by making use of the experiential knowledge that service users can bring to research. There is stronger evidence that service user involvement has an impact on the service users and researchers who are involved. However there are also potential drawbacks that should not be ignored including concerns about misdirection of research resources and tensions over differing agendas.
- *Current challenges*: At the present time there is a need to focus research efforts on service user involvement in research, to improve opportunities for comparison and analysis between research studies and internationally. Other challenges include establishing mechanisms to share existing learning, addressing representation issues, securing political and managerial support for involvement, making research more accessible and transparent, and developing more equal partnerships between service users and researchers.

Approaching service user involvement

Involving service users in research is a subject that has been described and approached in many ways. Take a moment to stop and think what the word *involvement* means to you. Why do you want to involve service users in research, or why do you want to be involved as a service user?

Your view of what involvement means is likely to be different from other people because there are so many ways of talking and thinking about service user involvement in research. Figure 1.1 illustrates some of the many terms and concepts that may be used to describe what involvement means. We will look at some of these concepts in more depth in the next chapter. Because it is common for different people to have different opinions about what involvement means it can be that expectations do not match and tensions may arise.

Some people think of involvement as a way of making sure that research addresses the types of questions that are important to service users. Some people think that it is a 'must-do' or something that they should be seen to be doing because policymakers and research commissioners say it is important. It might be described as being politically-correct, or PC. Other people think it is a way of getting service users' views heard or campaigning for improvements that service users want to see happen. Service users might say it is about making a contribution, giving something back by making the most of their experiences to change things for the better. Whilst other service users might say research is about gaining more understanding and control over their own lives. Of course people may agree or disagree with any of these different perspectives. They may have their own alternative view of what service user involvement in research means to them.

It is also important to remember that because of differences in cultural norms, professional disciplines and research traditions, some people may have never heard of service user involvement in research. There are also people who feel it does not relate to them and they are not a service user even if they are defined by professionals in this way. Differences in language can mean that service user involvement is more likely to be described as 'patient participation', 'public involvement', 'community participation', 'citizen engagement', or in other ways, depending on the context and who is speaking. Some of the conceptual differences between these terms are discussed in the next chapter.

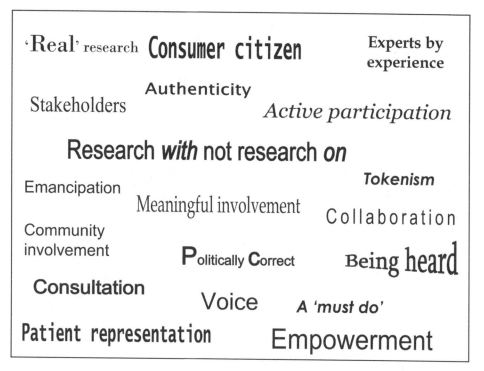

Figure 1.1   Key terms and concepts.

In essence 'service user involvement in research' means a situation where service users and researchers work together to design, undertake or evaluate research, rather than service users simply being the 'subjects' of the research. The phrase 'research *with* rather than research *on*' (INVOLVE 2004) captures this idea of an active relationship.

Sometimes service user involvement is thought of as an 'add on' to research studies. In this book we want to challenge that view because we see involvement as something that takes understanding, skill and expertise to initiate and to sustain. At the same time we also want to challenge the view that working with service users is a wholly 'good' thing for researchers to do. Service user involvement can provoke a whole range of responses and lead to many types of outcomes. There are both benefits and drawbacks to be aware of in the process.

Our take on service user involvement, and it is a view that many of the contributors to this book share, is that it is fundamentally about relationships. Our collective experience of working in nursing and healthcare research tells us that knowledge creation involves technical and social dimensions, which can also be personal and emotional. It is our belief that nursing and healthcare research should be about developing and improving upon existing knowledge to inform practice. It often means contesting what appears to be established concrete facts, looking for the gaps in *what* we know, but also the gaps in *how* we know.

As researchers we need to do more than create evidence and convey facts. We must also be concerned with how we make knowledge, including who we construct knowledge for.

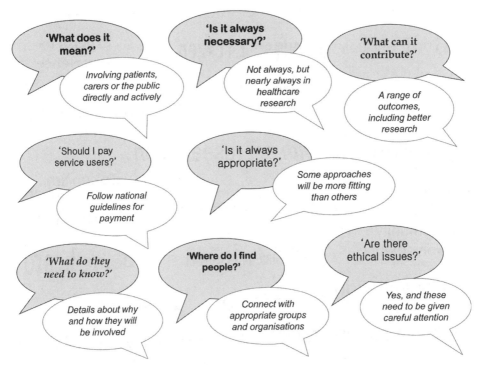

Figure 1.2   Common questions about service user involvement.

Working with service users helps to do that because it often involves reflecting, clarifying and revising the purpose and processes of the research. Involvement can bring researchers back to the fundamental questions that concern servicer users.

In this book we introduce a wide range of issues about service user involvement in research, such as the questions illustrated by Figure 1.2. Throughout the book we will keep four main questions in mind. The first question is *why*? Why should researchers involve service users? What are the purposes and the benefits? In the first section of the book – Preparing – we will explain some of the historical, social and political drivers behind service user involvement. We will show that service user involvement was not created over-night as a political idea, rather it emerged over the decades, growing out of beliefs, observations and ideas about how the quality of research practice might be improved and its outcomes be more relevant to healthcare practice and patients' needs.

The second question that we will keep in mind is *how?* How can researchers and service users work together? How can the process be successful and productive? In Chapter 3 we introduce models and a theoretical framework for thinking about service user involvement. Tools like this through the book will help you to think about, and learn from theory, so that you can make judgements about quality and impact. We also hope that the emphasis we have placed on reflective practice will help you to make the most of your own experiences for learning about how to improve ways of working.

The third question is *who?* We will look at issues about the types of service users that may become involved and consider the complex issues of representation and diversity, which so often arise in relation to service user involvement. We give particular attention to ways of involving seldom-heard groups in research (Chapter 7), bringing together practical advice about improving the accessibility of research, as well as looking at different ways in which service users and their representative organisations might undertake their own research (Chapter 8).

The fourth question is *when?* Above all, we want to convey the simple idea that relationships between researchers and service users do not just happen. They are forged and nurtured by people over time. We will explain why ideally service users should be involved from the outset of any research endeavour, and at all subsequent stages through the research.

To address these questions we put forward ideas from published research literature and relevant ongoing work. We have made use of information from health services research, mental health and learning disability research, child health, stroke, and sexual health. We have also asked researchers and service users to provide their own reflections and insights on the issues, and you will find these presented as case studies through the book.

Political and research contexts of involvement

A notable challenge for involving service users is ambiguity about the best ways to involve diverse groups of service users in different research contexts for different purposes – such as in research about treatments or care giving practices, identifying health needs, developing or planning of healthcare services, community health decision-making, 'basic' health research. It is also unclear how best to reflect the diverse and changing needs of different groups – such as patient, service user, client, relative, carer and caregiver perspectives, which may differ from the wider needs and preferences of the public. Diversity is therefore an important concept in relation to both the contexts of service user involvement, and to the professionals and service users it concerns. At the same time many of the challenges and opportunities of service user involvement are shared between professional groups and across disciplinary boundaries, such as a common interest in understanding patient experiences and translating these into improvements in healthcare.

This book focuses on service user involvement in the context of nursing and healthcare research but much of the story of development overlaps with trends towards service user involvement in the contexts of healthcare planning, delivery and development (Crawford et al. 2002). Some key events are outlined below and in the following section.

In 2000 in the UK, the organisation INVOLVE (at that time called Consumers in NHS Research) commissioned the organisation Folk.US to undertake a review of the research literature on service user involvement. The review sought together lessons from other fields and countries including social care, education, public health/health promotion, community development, housing/regeneration, agriculture/environment and development overseas. The resulting document, 'Small voices big noises' (Baxter et al. 2001) captured the main arguments in an accessible way and provided evidence to encourage research funders and sponsors to turn service user involvement into a reality. The report presents a number of lessons, which still have relevance today; these are:

- The importance of the political philosophy and context of research.
- The importance of shared values, mutual respect and trust, and common language in negotiations between partners about problems and solutions, as well as the need for clarity in the aims and expectations of research and in the roles and responsibilities for partners.
- The need for flexibility in research, including the methods used and the direction of the research.
- The need for flexibility of funding and the time allowed to undertake participatory projects.

The report reflects many other professional and academic debates going on at the turn of the millennium across the Western world. Such writings draw attention to the fact that it is important to enhance all areas of professional practice by ensuring that patients and the public are informed and involved in decisions that affect them.

In many Westernised countries it is now considered good practice to involve service users as part of the governance and regulation of health and social care research. For example, in the UK, requirements are laid out under the Research Governance Framework for Health and Social Care (Department of Health 2005) which advises that one aspect of a quality research culture should be that:

> Research is pursued with the active involvement of service users and carers including, where appropriate, those from hard-to-reach groups such as homeless people (p. 16).

Health and Social Care Act 2008 now consolidates much of the current legislation concerning the health service and health research. It awards increased support for service user involvement in health and social care research. Developments in other countries are explained later in the book (Chapter 11).

The following section looks at some of the key historical and social drivers of service user involvement, including challenges to medical authority, changing roles of patients in policy (patients as experts of their own health), political responses to research scandals, and the rise of consumerism and democratisation of public services.

Historical roots and social movements

It is important to appreciate that moves to involve service users in a wide-range of professional activities have come about because of the culmination of a series of historical events, rather than a one-off policy directive. Neither is service user involvement unique to nursing or healthcare research. Ideas about 'involvement' are also important in the context of the delivery of health services, service development and professional education. As illustrated by Figure 1.3, a series of historical events and social movements are what makes it possible for us to talk about service user involvement at this particular moment in time, and why it is possible for people to have contrary opinions about service user involvement. Here we will explain some of the key themes contributing to the rise of service user involvement in health and social care research.

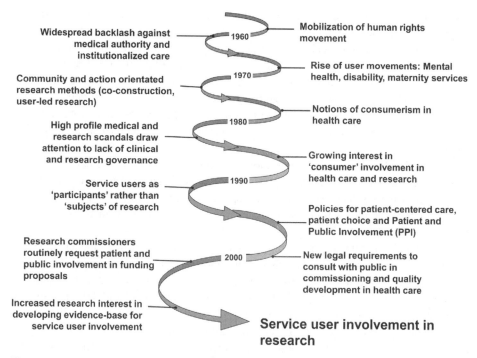

Widespread backlash against medical authority and institutionalized care

Community and action orientated research methods (co-construction, user-led research)

High profile medical and research scandals draw attention to lack of clinical and research governance

Service users as 'participants' rather than 'subjects' of research

Research commissioners routinely request patient and public involvement in funding proposals

Increased research interest in developing evidence-base for service user involvement

1960

1970

1980

1990

2000

Mobilization of human rights movement

Rise of user movements: Mental health, disability, maternity services

Notions of consumerism in health care

Growing interest in 'consumer' involvement in health care and research

Policies for patient-centered care, patient choice and Patient and Public Involvement (PPI)

New legal requirements to consult with public in commissioning and quality development in health care

Service user involvement in research

Figure 1.3 Historical events leading to service user involvement.

Challenges to medical authority

Long before there was talk of service user involvement in nursing or healthcare research there were concerns about whether public services work in the best interests of the public. In the 1950s, groups of patients across Westernised nations, particularly those with experience of institutionalised care, people with disabilities and mental health problems, began to question why they had no say in issues that affected them. The sharing and connection of personal stories about the unacceptability of publicly-funded institutions and professional practices gained support in the context of a wider public questioning of professional control over public matters (Entwistle et al. 1998).

In the 1960s, groups of the public took direct action on political issues. These trends are epitomised by the antiracism protests in the United States. Social welfare and human rights were key social issues internationally. Activists took up the notion of the 'healthcare consumer' and new consumer lobby groups gave individuals a position from which to campaign for particular health and service issues. The notion of 'public participation' first appears as a legal requirement in UK land use planning legislation in the 1960s (Regan 1978). Formal moves towards public participation in health services came considerably later with the introduction of the Patient's Charter for England (Department of Health 1996).

Changing roles of patients in policy

In the 1970s there was growing political recognition of public interests in public services. For example, cost containment at the macro level across healthcare systems involved setting prospective global budgets for hospitals, controls over hospital building and the acquisition of medical equipment, limits on doctor's fees and incomes, and restrictions on the numbers undertaking education and training. Governments began to encourage health service providers to deliver more consumer-focused and efficient care. These trends in health care supported the development of more community-focused and socially orientated approaches to research, such as Action Research and co-operative enquiry (Bryman 2001). In the UK, the women's lobby in maternity services and health consumer groups in general fed into new social movements which influenced research agendas and professional thinking about the social relations of research production (Oliver 1992). Early examples of lay involvement in the National Health Service focused on information and support, whether this was in maternity care, cancer care or health promotion (Oliver 1996). Even in these early stages the need for appropriate resourcing, training and support, and clarification of the role, nature and potential for service user involvement were known challenges (Oliver et al. 2001).

From the 1970s onwards mounting public unrest about political and professional decision-making escalated into a 'crisis of confidence' in how healthcare systems were being managed and run. Lobby groups and social networks began to directly challenge political decisions about health and social care. In the USA and UK, segregated communities, environmentalists and the disability movement used research findings to draw attention to everyday issues of discrimination and stigma in government policy. In relation to health services, ideas about patient empowerment and participation progressed through emancipatory and feminist debates surrounding healthcare practice and research (Williamson 2010).

Early articulations of service user involvement in health research appeared in the research literature on community-focused research in the late 1980s. Researchers using methods of co-construction and participation began to describe those involved in research as 'participants', rather than using the traditional term research 'subject'. The term subject was criticised for representing people as passive rather than active participants in the construction of knowledge. Hence, from the early 1990s onwards the literature more commonly uses the term 'participant', even if the nature of underlying power-relations remained the same.

User-led research

In the 1980s, emerging ideas about 'user-led' and 'user-controlled' research generated a new dimension to discussions about the purpose and impact of health research (Turner and Beresford 2005). Traditionally, health and social research had been approached as a way of attaining and transforming lay knowledge; however, interpretive and constructive approaches to research (discussed in Chapter 3) encourage the exploration of personal experience, for example using patients' experiences of health services to inform service development. User-led research focuses on research processes as much as research outcomes to enable service users to take part in carrying out research while gaining skills and confidence in the process (Faulkner and Thomas 2002). It aims to be inclusive and informative, ensuring that people who take part as research participants are kept fully informed of the results and of any action subsequently taken. User-controlled research is research which is actively controlled, directed and managed by service users and is accountable to them (Beresford 2009). Service users decide on the issues and questions to be looked at, as well as the way the research is designed, planned and written up. Some service users make a distinction between the term 'user-controlled' and 'user-led' research, as they feel that user-led research has a vaguer meaning (see Chapter 8).

Consumerism

In the late 1980s/early 1990s, continued drives for efficiency and responsiveness to end-users introduced market-like mechanisms in the health service and management reforms as well as budgetary incentives. In the UK, political interests looked towards consumer-ism and introducing new types of internal market forces to the NHS (Potter 1988). Consumerism was heralded as a way of reframing public and professional relationships, by applying principles of access, choice, information, redress and representation to public services. Consumerism brought with it the broad reawakening of the idea of participation and a new emphasis on the rights and responsibilities of citizens. Some researchers talked about top-down 'consumerist' approaches to involvement in contrast with empowerment (Barnes and Walker 1996). Beresford (2002) developed this line of thinking and argued that top-down politically/managerially controlled service user involvement had subsumed a bottom-up lay ideology of democratic empowerment.

Democratisation of public services

In the mid-1990s policymakers across Westernised nations were attempting to shift the focus of governance towards new forms of co-production with other agencies and with citizens themselves through partnerships and community involvement. Policy discourses began to construct multiple public identities through the use of particular terms, for example, 'active citizenship', 'confident consumers', and 'expert patients', who are 'more responsible, more informed and more actively involved in choices about their own health'. Greater spending and commissioning authority was awarded to local health bodies and public and private partnerships were encouraged. Under these conditions patient satisfaction became more important to policymakers, healthcare managers, practitioners and service users, but this has brought its own problems of defining what a diverse range of service users want and how patient experiences of care can be measured.

Public responses to professional scandals

Despite trends towards greater recognition of public interests in public services and greater emphasis on efficiency and responsiveness to service users, arguably the most significant drivers for service user involvement have been concerns about safety in health services and health research. From the late 1960s a wave of scandals surfaced across the Western world about specific treatments, such as the prescription of thalidomide to preg-nant women. Medical scandals drew attention to the lack of restrictions around medical research on patients. For example, in the UK the child deaths in heart surgery at Bristol (Bristol Royal Infirmary Inquiry 2001) and the retention of children's body parts for research at Alder Hey Hospital in Liverpool (The Alder Hey Inquiry 2001) were the ultimate trigger for political action towards greater public involvement in health care. Patient safety adds pace and a new urgency to the imperative of involvement. Later in the book we will examine the main legal and ethical issues in relation to service user involvement in research, such as data protection and confidentiality requirements (Chapter 4).

At the present time governments are encouraging citizens to take greater responsibility for their own health, through initiatives such as health promotion campaigns, health checks and personal health insurance. Service users are no longer thought of as passive recipients of health care, they are considered active participants in their own health and well-being. In the UK the new coalition government, and the challenges of quality and productivity, are likely to bring a new stance to the issues of involvement.

Perspectives of service user involvement

As we have already seen, the idea of service user involvement in research is made up of many concepts and issues. You should also be aware that different professional groups and disciplines may hold different views about what service user involvement means and how it should be carried out. For example, there are different stances to involvement between the medical professions, therapists and social work. Figure 1.4 illustrates some of the different perspectives that might be brought to service user involvement in research. Within each of these perspectives there can be disagreement and uncertainty about what service user involvement is or should be.

From the perspective of research commissioners, incorporating service user involvement into a research study can be a deciding factor in the award of research funding. In the UK context research funders ask that applications for funding should show a 'commitment' to service user involvement. The National Institute for Health Research is one example of a funding body that requests information about how service users will be involved in the proposed research. Researchers applying for grants need to show they are engaging seriously with service user involvement and to explain how this will be undertaken. Often research funders, including charitable organisations, want to see that service user involvement is well thought through and is appropriate to the proposed research. It means that there should be adequate planning, attention to ethical issues, and that involvement should be sufficiently costed into the requested budget. At the present time most research funders do not formally audit service user involvement but they may stipulate that involvement work is written-up as part of the project report.

Researchers are known to hold very different views about the purpose and value of service user involvement. Their views may be influenced by research structures and systems that inform how they work, such as funding systems, ethical review processes, research governance structures, and their employing research institutions. Researcher's opinions of service user involvement may also be influenced by the research systems they work within, such as the research methods they use, favoured theories, concepts and strategies. Later in the book we will look at how different approaches to involvement have tended to emerge in different research contexts and areas of research practice (Chapter 3).

Although there is growing public interest in service user involvement, at the present time there is very little information about what service users expect when they agree, or decide, to become involved in research. Service users may see research as an opportunity to

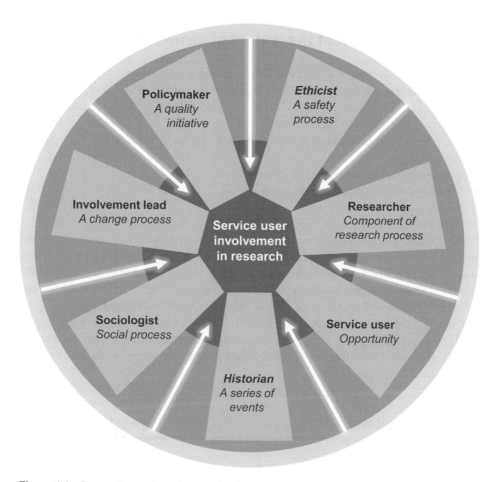

Figure 1.4   Perspectives of service user involvement in research.

improve health or social care services, even though research can sometimes seem like a long and indirect way of bringing change. Some service users talk about wanting to 'give something back' to a health or social system that has helped them or family members, sometimes described as 'reciprocity' (Crighton et al. 2002). Some people want to do something to improve the situation for other people that are, or may go through, what they have experienced. This has been called 'altruism' or being 'altruistic' (Entwistle et al. 1998).

Other service users may see research as a chance to find out information about their condition or to meet people who have had similar health experiences as them. Some people want to develop their skills or knowledge, towards entering into education or employment, or as a way of earning money. The motives for wanting to become involved in research are as diverse as those held by professional researchers. As a minimum, good practice guidelines emphasise that service users should expect to be given sufficient information about their involvement in the research, to be respected, to be involved in ways that suit them, and for their contributions to the research to be acknowledged (Telford et al. 2004). These and other aspects of quality involvement are discussed in Chapter 9.

What is known about the impact of involvement?

A common question that is asked is what service user involvement contributes to research – what impact does it have? It is an important question that encompasses issues about the:

- Extent to which service user involvement is being undertaken across the research community,
- Scope and nature of service user's influence, and
- Types of outcomes that can be achieved.

We will look at these issues of impact in Chapter 10.

We do know that interest in service user involvement is growing internationally. At the present time many research organisations and networks are engaging service users in new ways. As a recent review shows, there are numerous strong accounts to suggest that the quality of research studies can be improved by making use of the experiential knowledge (Staley 2009). We will look at some of the evidence in Part III of the book.

Current thinking is that service user involvement in research can have a range of different types of impacts. Figure 1.5 illustrates what some of these impacts can be, including potential benefits and drawbacks. Until recently the tendency has been to focus

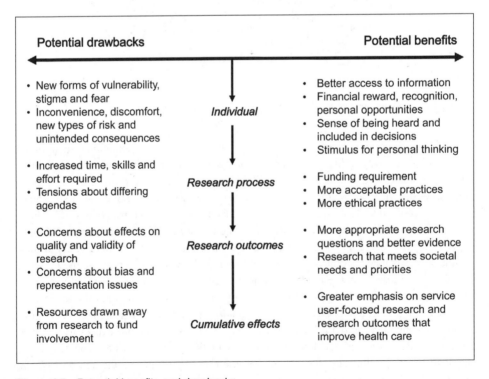

Figure 1.5   Potential benefits and drawbacks.

on producing evidence that service user involvement is beneficial to individuals involved and to the research, rather than creating a balanced view of what works, for whom, in what circumstances (INVOLVE 2009).

Current challenges

At the present time there is a need to focus research efforts on service user involvement in research, to improve opportunities for comparison and analysis between research studies and internationally. The development of programmes of research has been hindered so far because relatively few focal areas have emerged. Where there is a cluster of activity, for example, on involving children in research, more could be done to spread learning from previous studies to address recurrent practical and methodological issues (Staley 2009). The PIN project (Patient and public involvement in nursing, midwifery and health visiting research) drew attention to the fact that current definitions and models of service user involvement in research (discussed in Chapter 2) tend to direct attention towards interactions between service users and professional researchers at research project level. In so doing, they fail to take into consideration the wider contextual issues of how research cultures and values construct, influence and limit such interactions (Smith et al. 2008).

A further challenge is sharing existing learning. Some areas of healthcare research have benefited from knowledge spread through strong networks such as mental health, disability research and some areas of cancer research. In the UK the work of the INVOLVE Support Unit has included producing guidelines for commissioners, researchers and the public on involvement in research grant applications, peer reviewing applications and research commissioning and supporting an online discussion forum (www.invo.org.uk/forum). Clearly research from outside the specific field of research practice and from other research disciplines, including research on participation in the delivery of health services and social care research, could be used more to inform thinking about service user involvement in nursing and healthcare research.

There is also a related need to know how representation is played out in different research settings with different types of service users (Boote et al. 2002). Representation issues continue to be a challenge and barrier to service user involvement in research. Some of the reasons why are discussed in the next chapter.

A further challenge is how policymakers, research commissioners and different research communities can support and develop service user involvement, without overly controlling or bureaucratising the process. To date, a very small proportion of research is specifically led by service users or carers (Turner and Beresford 2005). While research commissioners are now more open to funding user-led research and consumer and voluntary organisations have funded research led by patient-researchers, very little is known about the leadership and influencing role of service users. We will look at these issues in more depth in Chapter 8.

Many researchers are concerned about how research can be more accessible and transparent to those it is about. Some advances have been made in raising awareness about using accessible language, for example, making sure scientific terms and abbreviations are explained in clear language and that research reports contain lay summaries. Other issues that research teams face are being clear about processes of decision-making, explaining different interests and underlying intentions by making such information available for discussion and debate with those service users who are involved.

A further challenge is how to achieve more equal partnerships between service users and researchers, which allow for the fact that each will have different types of contributions to make and responsibilities to fulfil. At the present time professional researchers generally hold responsibility for research governance and ethics even when service users are involved in managing the research. Furthermore, concepts of professional responsibility including duty of care and informed consent guide understandings about who is accountable for the research. At the same time new forms of responsibility have emerged – such as peer-support and service user training – which may not currently be recognised by existing accountability structures. Alternatively, service users who are involved may see working in partnership as an issue of getting the practical aspects of engagement right.

Key principles for practice

- There are multiple notions of service user involvement in research, but in general it means the active and direct participation of patients, carers or members of the public in research and its associated activities.
- Across many Westernised nations there is strong political interest in engaging the public more actively in a wide-range of professional areas of working.
- There are longstanding historical and ethical reasons behind service user involvement in research.
- Service user involvement should be appropriate to the research, there should be adequate planning and budgeting, and service users should be given sufficient information, be involved in ways that suit them and they should be respected and acknowledged.
- Although service user involvement can improve the quality of research studies there are also potential drawbacks that should not be ignored including use of research resources and research agendas.
- Service user involvement in research is not without its ethical, methodological and practical challenges. These require further research and learning.

References

Barnes, M. and Walker, A. (1996) Consumerism versus empowerment: a principled approach to the involvement of older service users. *Policy and Politics*, 24 (4): 375–94.

Baxter, L., Thorne, L., and Mitchell, A. (2001) *Small Voices Big Noises. Lay Involvement in Health Research: Lessons from Other Fields*. Eastleigh: INVOLVE.

Beresford, P. (2002) User involvement in health research and evaluation: liberation or regulation? *Social Policy & Society*, 1 (2): 95–105.

Beresford, P. (2009) User-controlled research. In: Wallcraft, J. Schrank, B. and Amering, M. (eds) *Handbook of Service User Involvement in Mental Health Research*. Chichester: Wiley-Blackwell.

Boote, J., Telford, R., and Cooper, C. (2002) Consumer involvement in health research: a review and research agenda. *Health Policy*, 61 (2): 213–36.

Bristol Royal Infirmary Inquiry (2001) *The Inquiry into the Management of Care of Children Receiving Complex Heart Surgery at the Bristol Royal Infirmary*. London: Department of Health.

Bryman, A. (2001) *Social Research Methods*. Oxford: Oxford University Press.

Crawford, M., Rutter, D., Manley, C., Weaver, T., Bhui, K., Fulop, N., and Tyrer, P. (2002) Systematic review of involving patients in the planning and development of health care. *British Medical Journal*, 325: 1263–5.

Crighton, M.H., Goldberg, A.N., and Kagan, S.H. (2002) Reciprocity for patients with head and neck cancer participating in an instrument development project. *Oncology Nursing Society – Online Exclusive/Research Brief*, 29: 10.

Department of Health (1996) *The Patient's Charter & You. A Charter for England*. London: Department of Health.

Department of Health (2005) *Research Governance Framework for Health and Social Care*, 2nd edn. London: Department of Health.

Department of Health (2008) *Health and Social Care Act*, Section 242. London: Department of Health.

Entwistle, V., Renfrew, M., Yearley, S., Forrester, J., and Lamont, T. (1998) Lay perspectives: advantages for health research. *British Medical Journal*, 316: 463–6.

Faulkner, A. and Thomas, P. (2002) User-led research and evidence based medicine. *The British Journal of Psychiatry*, 180: 1–3.

INVOLVE (2004) *Involving Consumers in Research and Development in the NHS. Briefing Notes for Researchers,* 2nd edn. Eastleigh: INVOLVE. (Available from: www.invo.org.uk)

INVOLVE (2009) *The Impact of Public Involvement on Research. A Discussion Paper from the INVOLVE Evidence, Knowledge and Learning Working Group*. Eastleigh: INVOLVE.

Oliver, M. (1992) Changing the social relations of research production. *Disability, Handicap and Society*, 7 (2): 101–14.

Oliver, S. (1996) The progress of lay involvement in the NHS Research and Development Programme. *Journal of Evaluation in Clinical Practice*, 2 (4): 273–80.

Oliver, S., Milne, R., Bradburn, J., Buchanan, P., Kerridge, L., Walley, T., and Gabbay, J. (2001) Involving consumers in a needs-led research programme: A pilot project. *Health Expectations*, 4 (1): 18–28.

Potter, J. (1988) Consumerism and the public sector: how well does the coat fit? *Public Administration*, 66: 149–64.

Regan, D. (1978) The pathology of British land use planning. *Local Government Studies*, 1743-9388, 4 (2): 3–23.

Smith, E., Ross, F., Donovan, S., Manthorpe, J., Brearley, S., Sitzia, J., and Beresford, P. (2008) Service user involvement in nursing, midwifery and health visiting research: a review of evidence and practice. *International Journal of Nursing Studies*, 45 (2): 298–315.

Staley, K. (2009) *Exploring Impact: Public Involvement in NHS, Public Health and Social Care Research*. Eastleigh: INVOLVE.

Telford, R., Boote, J., and Cooper, C. (2004) What does it mean to involve consumers successfully in NHS research? A consensus study. *Health Expectations*, 7 (3): 209–20.

The Alder Hey Inquiry (2001) *The Report of the Royal Liverpool Children's Inquiry*. London: Department of Health.

Turner, P. and Beresford, P. (2005) *User controlled research: its meanings and potential. Final Report*. INVOLVE, Shaping our lives and the centre for citizen participation, Brunel University. Eastleigh: INVOLVE.

Williamson, C. (2010) *Towards the Emancipation of Patients. Patients' Experiences and the Patient Movement*. Bristol: The Policy Press.

Chapter 2

Concepts

Key summary points

- *Service users*: The concept of 'service user' encompasses a wide range of individuals, groups and organisations. It is most often used to mean patients or clients of health services but it can also mean people who do not access services or the potential recipients of health care. 'Carers' are sometimes included under the term service user but they should be perceived as having a distinct and separate perspective from those that they care for.
- *Involvement*: The concept of 'involvement' is closely associated with 'being included', 'participating' and 'having a say' in the issues. The concept is problematic because it implies a situation where service users are invited into professional research worlds, yet service users may undertake their own research, or contest existing research practices. It does not adequately reflect the fact that service user involvement can extend beyond involvement in a particular research study or programme, for example in reviewing or evaluating research.
- *Representation*: Notions of 'representation' can be a point of confusion because there are different concepts and it can sometimes be unclear what or who service users are being asked to represent.
- *Experiential knowledge*: Service users have firsthand real life experiences that they can bring to the research, which has been called 'experiential knowledge'.
- *Empowerment*: The concept of 'empowerment' is a positive or supportive process which may involve participation or mutual decision-making and freedom to make choices and accept responsibility.
- *Participation*: The term 'participation' is generally used to describe a collaborative process of working together, where service users and researchers respect the different types of skills, knowledge and abilities that each can bring to the research. It can also mean taking a shared approach to decision-making about the research.
- *Models of involvement*: Authors have developed or made use of models to help explain the types of relationships between service users and researchers in research. These include a ladder of participation, levels of involvement (consultation, collaboration, control), and a continuum of participation. In practice, how service user involvement is played out in any particular study is likely to change over time as researchers and service users become more aware of each other's strengths and contributions to the research.

Handbook of Service User Involvement in Nursing and Healthcare Research, First Edition.
Elizabeth Morrow, Annette Boaz, Sally Brearley and Fiona Ross.
© 2012 Elizabeth Morrow, Annette Boaz, Sally Brearley and Fiona Ross.
Published 2012 by Blackwell Publishing Ltd.

• *A theoretical framework for approaching service user involvement in research*: A helpful way of understanding service user involvement in research is to think of it as having four interrelated components: context, methods, roles and outcomes. This helps to put the issues together and see how they are related. These four components are also potential areas for personal and professional learning.

Service users

Issues of terminology are important for understanding what service user involvement in research is and how it is understood in the literature and research practice. Readers should keep in mind that the language is developing rapidly in this field and different terms are used to mean different things in different research and healthcare contexts, and internationally (see Chapter 11).

From the early 1970s onwards researchers using community- and action-orientated research methods began to describe those involved in research as 'participants', rather than using the more traditional term research 'subject'. The term subject was criticised for representing people as passive rather than active participants in the construction of knowledge (Beresford and Croft 1996). Hence, from the early 1990s onwards the health and social care research literature more commonly uses the term 'participant' and greater attention was being paid to the nature of underlying power-relations between the researcher and the researched. In health service development, the meaning and mechanisms of patient participation were also being debated (Cahill 1996).

Entering the new millennium the language took a new turn towards 'consumer involvement' in research. This trend reflects politically driven debates about the introduction of consumer-driven mechanisms of choice and demand in to the provision of health care (previously discussed in Chapter 1). Although still sometimes used in policy and research publications, the term 'consumer' has been perceived as being a politically derived term at odds with values of partnership and inclusion (Beresford 2005). More recently the term 'public involvement' has begun to appear in international literatures, reflecting a widespread growing interest in engaging the public in decisions about health care (Beresford 2007).

Clearly being a 'patient' and being a 'participant in research' involves very different things. It also demands different types of responses from professionals. Confusion of the two identities can lead to profound misunderstandings about what is appropriate (Lidz and Applebaum 2002). For example, a patient may discuss their health status in great detail during a clinical intervention but in the context of participating in a research study they may not wish to disclose or discuss their personal health status. On the other hand, the professional may not feel it is appropriate for them to be approached as a clinician, for example for personal medical or treatment advice, when they are undertaking the research. This is a particular issue to be aware of where clinical researchers are working with their own patients in research studies. It is best to think of these as two different types of relationships and to talk through the differences with the person concerned in confidence to establish what is and is not acceptable.

Box 2.1   Barnes and Wistow's (1994) classification of 'service users'

- *Voluntary and involuntary users* – indicating the degree of willingness with which individuals engage with services.
- *Short-term and long-term users* – is the relationship concluded when a specific outcome has been achieved, or is the service offered one which has to be sustained throughout a lengthy period?
- *Individuals as allies or competitors* – do users of services identify themselves as having common interests? Do they regard themselves as competitors for scarce resources?
- *Individuals and group interests* – is the service provided and received on an individual or collective basis?
- *Actual and potential users* – service user should not be equated with the existence of a need. There are many reasons why someone may not use services, although he or she could be considered to have needs which services are intended to meet.
- *Users and carers* – carers may have needs in their own right and they may be direct users of services. However, their needs should be distinguished from the needs of those to whom they provide a service.
- *Users and citizens* – all citizens are potential users of services, and accountability to citizens is an essential characteristic of public services. However, the interests of current users of services may be seen to conflict with those of citizens who are not users.

All role titles, such as 'nurse', 'patient' and 'service user', have positioning power. For some people they feel the term 'service user' defines them according to something they are not – a 'service provider'. They argue that it is too simplistic to see the world as being divided into users and providers. Some people feel it is more fitting to call themselves a 'survivor', or to emphasise the term can mean more than one thing (Turner and Beresford 2005). Describing who 'service users' are in detail can help to convey the diversity of individual people involved in any one research study or programme (see Barnes and Wistow's 1994 classification, Box 2.1). Providing such detail also helps to acknowledge some of the differences in the way people use services.

A further issue to be aware of is that the term 'user' is often used in policy and research publications to mean those *who may use research*, those *whom research is about*, and those *it might affect*. Figure 2.1 illustrates some of the individuals and groups who may be considered 'service users'. However, carers should be thought of as being distinctly different from service users, as discussed below.

A carer is someone who, without payment, provides help and support to a partner, child, relative, friend or neighbour, who could not manage without their help. This could be due to age, physical or mental illness, addiction or disability. They may provide care occasionally or on a full-time basis. A carer may be one of several people who do things to help a person to cope with their health problems, or they may be the only person that they trust. Young carers are children or young people under the age of 18 who carry out significant caring tasks for another person. As a group of people 'carers' are not the same as patients or the general public. Although carers also use health services and may need health or social care support themselves, their experiences are different from that of the people they care for. Carers have their own expectations, needs and opinions. They may call attention to issues or deficiencies in treatment and service delivery because of their particular view of what is important. They may also undertake 'carer-led' research (see Chapters 5 and 8).

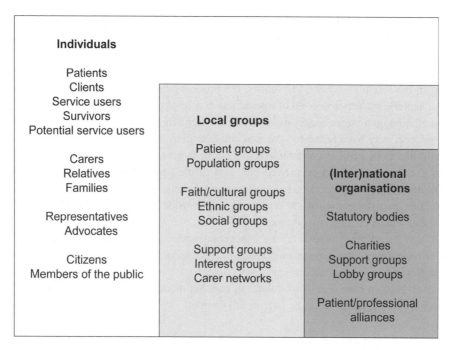

Figure 2.1   Individuals and groups who may be considered 'service users'.

Paid 'care workers', residential and hospital carers are usually considered to be staff rather than carers. The terms 'formal' and 'informal carer' are used to make this distinction in health care. Many carers do not like this terminology, as 'informal' caring implies that the roles of carers and carer workers are essentially similar except that one receives pay and the other doesn't. However there are enormous differences. Paid workers can choose their job and their client group, and they have conditions of service including set hours and holidays. Carers may not feel they have such choices and may see caring as part of their relationship. They may be supporting their person out of love, family responsibility and other loyalties. Living with someone who requires care can be tiring, worrying, stressful, upsetting and emotionally draining, but it can also be rewarding and fulfilling.

Involvement

The concept of involvement has been debated extensively in the research literature. Most authors suggest that the term carries intrinsic associations with 'being included', 'participating' and 'having a say' in the issues (Cayton 2002). Other authors are more critical of the concept because it implies a situation where service users are brought into professional research worlds. Furthermore, it overlooks the fact that service users may lead, control or undertake research themselves (Turner and Beresford 2005). Involvement does not capture the fact that service user involvement often extends beyond a particular research study or programme. Service users' views may not condone or support the research but they may still have an interest in it, for example involvement in reviewing or evaluating research.

'Involvement' also implies that service users are being invited to be an active participant in the research, whereas in reality, the process can be tokenistic (defined later in this chapter) or a very low level of interaction may be experienced, for example minimal consultation on a minor aspect of the research (Beresford 2005). In such circumstances researchers may have failed to take into consideration the ways in which service users would like to be involved or attention has not been given to service users' views about how the research should be carried out. Part of the problem is that researchers have different understandings of what involvement means. Some would see information giving as involvement whilst others would only consider working in collaboration with service users to count as involvement.

A way to address some of these conceptual uncertainties is for research teams to describe in detail what type of involvement is planned and to document the service user activities that have been undertaken (see Chapter 9). It can also be beneficial for research teams to explain how their work relates to existing models of service user involvement, which we will go on to describe later in this chapter.

Representation

The terms 'representation' and 'representative' have many meanings but are often used when describing who can, or should represent the views of service users.

In relation to service user involvement in research there is little agreement about the conceptual meaning of representation because of the wide range of people who may be described as being service users. In the past, the argument that service user involvement is not representative has been used to devalue, exclude and disempower service users (Beresford and Campbell 1994). This is why it is important to understand that representation has different meanings.

A 'representative' can be someone who is elected by means of a democratic process. For example, if a person is voted onto a patient's council through a ballot. In this approach it is important to be clear about the criteria for nomination, election and the 'community' that are being represented. Otherwise it could be questioned whether it is fair for a particular person to be a representative, and to be clear about when someone else should have a chance to take on the role.

Being 'representative' could also mean that a person has been selected on the basis of statistical representation, so that they can be considered typical of others who share similar experiences. This approach does not work well in the case of the representation of service user experiences or views because everyone's perspectives and experiences are unique. The views of statistically representative samples of people may not always provide the most appropriate form of information about health services or health issues. For example, in community and service development projects that aim to improve service user access to health services, it may be necessary to target particular groups because of their age, ethnicity or religious background. It may also be inappropriate to define a

---

Box 2.2   Forms of representation

- *Democratic representation* – 'One person one vote', equally weighted voting.
- *Proportional representation* – The use of shared or weighted votes to represent different groups.
- *Statistical representation* – Could include selection, randomisation or controlled samples.
- *Representational membership* – Nominated or elected individuals represent the views of their candidacy.
- *Representation by someone who is 'typical' of others* – An individual is nominated or identified because they are thought to share similar experiences or characteristics as others.
- *Dispositional representation* – Individuals become or adopt representative roles by virtue of their job/organisational membership.
- *Representation of shared interests (radicalism, lobbying)* – Self-nominated representatives form groups on the basis of their shared interests.
- *Representation of self* – Personal image, interests and decisions.

'sample' of people in the context of aiming to achieve more active forms of participation that recognise service users' unique experiences and personal qualities.

Concerns have been raised that undue weight may be given to the views of just a few, perhaps isolated individuals. It is also important to recognise that the decision to become involved is a two way process and there will be personal reasons for why individuals may choose to become involved. Issues of representation need to be considered in the light of the fact that often service users' perspectives are not represented at all in research. A more balanced argument is that although a service user cannot be representative a service user perspective can be represented (Russell et al. 2002).

The concept of representing the 'user voice' has been influential in conceptualising interactions between patients and healthcare professionals and health service organisations. For example, Lohan and Coleman (2005) show that in relation to sexual health service development, professional codes of practice (confidentiality, consent, contact tracing) contribute to the absence of the lay voice. Voice is often approached as an ethical issue for service user perspectives to be represented in professional practice or as a question of overcoming barriers to 'being heard'. Such a perspective aligns with a concept of representation where self-nominated representatives form lobby groups for the purpose of formulating and expressing their shared interests. Other researchers have asked exactly what the 'user voice' signifies and to what purpose the 'voice' will be put (Seymour and Skilbeck 2002).

Concerns about 'being representative' link to the concern that some service users are involved more than others and this can mean individuals become 'professionalised' to research environments (Rhodes et al. 2001). One approach is to involve new service users by 'refreshing' the membership of groups (Davies et al. 2006). Yet service users may feel better able to contribute when they have gained considerable knowledge and experience about the research. It also takes time to build up trust and good working relationships which are not easily replaced (Ross et al. 2005). In practice, it should be made clear to service users the forms of representation that the research team is employing (such as those summarised in Box 2.2) as well as who, what and which type of perspectives service users are being asked to represent.

As new forms of research have developed issues of representation are not escaped, they are manifest in new ways. For example, in the context of user-controlled research representation becomes an issue of identifying shared interests and how best to generate knowledge that will lead to change.

Experiential knowledge

We tend to take it for granted that everyone has the same understanding of what knowledge is. Knowledge is often perceived as something fixed that can be learnt, or known such as facts or evidence. However, what knowledge is has been debated by many philosophers and theorists for a long time. The study of the nature and scope of knowledge is called epistemology.

Knowledge can be classified according to what it is about, for example the clinical indicators of stroke, or the procedure for hip replacement. Knowledge can also be classified according to how it has been constructed, for example using clinical observations or a quantitative survey of patient's views. Most knowledge in the real world is a combination of many forms of knowledge – for example, professional, social and experiential knowledge may all be used during a consultation between a nurse and a patient to make an assessment of care needs. Some of these forms of knowledge are illustrated by Figure 2.2.

The concept of 'experiential knowledge' is sometimes used in relation to service user involvement to mean knowledge that is based in firsthand real life experiences (Beresford 2003), or 'lay perspectives'. Another term that is sometimes used to describe such knowledge is 'authentic'. Experiential knowledge is thought of as being distinctly different

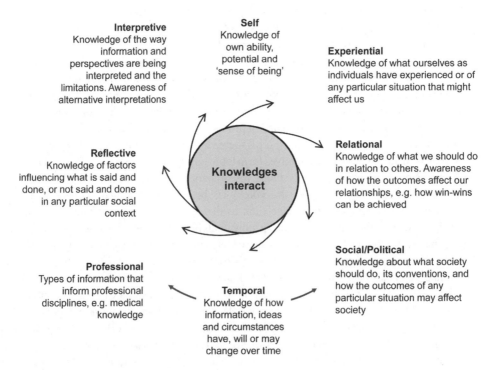

Figure 2.2   Types of knowledge.

from other types of knowledge that healthcare professionals or researchers might draw upon. The concept of experiential knowledge has been debated extensively in the research literature. The main points of debate can be summarised as follows:

- Debates about the usefulness of lay perspectives (e.g. Entwistle et al. 1998; Glasby and Littlechild 2001; Marshall et al. 2007).
- The standing of lay knowledge compared to other types of knowledge (Pawson et al. 2003; Popay and Williams 1998).
- The appropriateness of particular research methods for accessing such information (e.g. Edwards 2000; Edwards and Titchen 2003; Ryan et al. 2001).
- Issues about ownership of lay knowledge, which traditionally has been with those who have skills and ability to produce research evidence (Entwistle et al. 2002; Glasby and Beresford 2006).

The process of finding or generating new knowledge is generally thought of as research. For example, in the introduction to this book we explained that in our view nursing and healthcare research is about the generation of knowledge to inform practice, education, management and policy development that relates to these professional roles. In relation to service user involvement in research much of the debate in this field has focused on questioning dominant concepts of scientific evidence and the means of production of such evidence (Glasby and Beresford 2006). Evidence-based practice (EBP) advocates using the best available evidence from research, along with patient preferences and clinical experience, when making decisions (Cullum 2000). 'Best evidence' is often thought of as evidence generated by means of the randomised controlled trial (RCT) (Rothwell 2005). However, EBP is not just about the application of research trial generated knowledge in the clinical arena, but also involves clinicians' judgements and patients' values (Sackett et al. 1996). In Chapter 12, we will look in more depth at how service user involvement in research can help to enhance EBP.

Empowerment

The concept of empowerment is often used in nursing practice, education, research and health promotion to mean a positive or supportive process. It usually refers to 'a partnership valuing self and others, mutual decision-making and freedom to make choices and accept responsibility' (Rodwell 1996). The term may be used to describe a personal experience of being involved in research – 'feeling empowered' – as well as other types of activities. It is sometimes used to describe the aims of a research study – 'to empower' – or as an outcome of service user involvement – 'empowerment'.

Empowerment has also been perceived of as a political idea, to which the ownership of power, inequalities of power and the acquisition and redistribution of power are central. Ideas about empowerment through participation emphasise people gaining control over public services, influencing services to meet their needs, and so having more control over their lives (Rodgers 1994).

Concepts of empowerment can be quite problematic because whilst the term carries inherent meaning it suggests that power is a finite entity that can be gained or attained

(Bhavnani 1990). In reality power is manifest through a whole range of social values, processes and interactions (Clegg 1989). Another conceptual problem is that being empowered (with the help and intervention of others) and emancipating oneself is not the same thing (Mercer 2002). This makes it difficult to judge whether a person has been empowered or not, as they may not feel they have been empowered or that they gained power through their own actions.

Despite these conceptual uncertainties, in recent years the idea of 'research as empowerment' has also been taken up by the commercial sector. For example, the market and public opinion research agency MORI formed a Participation Unit with the objective of engaging people in a dialogue and to 'empower the researched to become the researcher' (Christopoulos and Rose 2006). The organisation began to employ new, more sophisticated techniques such as pyramid interviewing (training members of the community to interview others), and bifocal groups (discussion groups involving people with contrasting experiences, e.g., healthcare providers and service users). Later in the book the section on quality experiences of involvement (Chapter 9) helps to take forward discussions about empowerment by examining how individuals, both service users and professional researchers, make judgements about research practice and enact these ideas through their own thinking and conduct.

Participation

The concept of patient participation is widely used in contemporary nursing, midwifery and health visiting practice. It forms part of the language of professional practice and is generally thought of as a way of enhancing decision-making, for example about health choices or treatment options. In healthcare delivery patient participation can enrich a patient's quality of life by allowing them to express their personal preferences and priorities for care (Coulter 1999).

The concept of participation also emerges through wider health and social care policies where it has acquired new meaning and characteristics. In the context of political thinking participation is more likely to mean the responsibility of citizens to be an informed and active participant in their own health. For example, partnership between healthcare providers and the public is also a strong feature of public health promotion, most notably in quitting smoking campaigns and patient partnerships for improved healthcare associated infection control. Policies to encourage individual citizens to become more involved in decisions and choices about their own health have influenced thinking about participation in other contexts including management, education and research (Needham 2003).

In relation to service user involvement in health research, 'participation' can mean anything from being informed about the research to a collaborative process of working together. The terms involvement and participation are often used interchangeably. In the UK current research policy and research commissioning guidelines suggest that the safety, acceptability and relevance of research, can be improved through public participation. Whilst this may or may not be true, the process of participation in research means that service users and researchers are more likely to understand and respect the different types of skills, knowledge and abilities that each can bring to the research. Participation is often associated with notions of working in partnership and taking a shared approach to decision-making about the research. Whilst participation is likely to be interpreted as service users 'having a say' about the issues, it is more likely that partnership is seen as a process of working towards mutual benefit through discussion and negotiation. Conceptualisations of public participation, such as the models discussed in the following section, support the idea that different levels and forms of participation are appropriate in different circumstances of public decision-making and healthcare contexts (Brooks 2006).

Models of involvement

A ladder of participation

Perhaps the most influential and frequently reproduced model is Sheri Arnstein's ladder of citizen participation (Arnstein 1969), which describes a continuum of activities from manipulation to citizen control. This model was developed in the USA as a result of heated controversy over issues of citizen participation, and in particular the involvement of the poor in federal social programmes. Arnstein argued that 'there is a critical difference between going through the empty ritual of participation and having the real power needed to affect the outcome of the process'. She identified that roadblocks to achieving 'genuine' levels of participation lie on both sides (state and citizen) including racism, paternalism and resistance to power distribution, inadequacies of socioeconomic infrastructure and knowledge base, as well as difficulties of organising representative and accountable citizen's groups. Figure 2.3 illustrates how a ladder of participation might be perceived in relation to nursing and healthcare research.

Tritter and McCallum (2006) suggest that Arnstein's model, by solely emphasising power, limits effective responses to the challenges of involving service users in healthcare

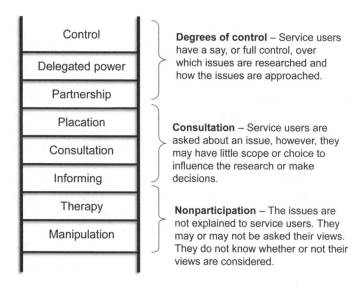

Figure 2.3   A ladder of participation.

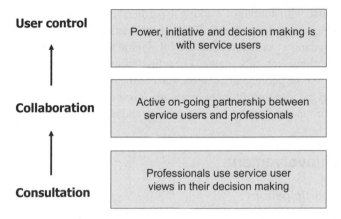

Figure 2.4   Levels of service user control.

contexts and undermines the potential of the involvement process. This is because such an emphasis on power assumes that it has a common meaning for service users, providers and policymakers and ignores the existence of different relevant forms of knowledge and expertise. It also fails to recognise that for some service users, participation itself may be a goal. These authors argue that for service user involvement to be better understood models must be sufficiently broad to acknowledge the value of the process and the diversity of knowledge and experience of both professionals and service users. Tritter and McCallum propose that a mosaic is a better metaphor for service user involvement as it illustrates the relationship between horizontal and vertical accountability and enables involvement to be mapped and monitored.

Levels of control

Service users are sometimes perceived as having different roles in the research that relate to levels of control in the research process (INVOLVE 2004). A well known classification is consultation, collaboration and user-control (Figure 2.4). Consultation with service users is sometimes described as a low level of involvement as the service provider or researcher keeps control of the overall agenda, or makes use of service user contributors views to inform their decision-making (Sweeney and Morgan 2009). Collaboration is a more active partnership between service users and researchers, where decision-making power is shared. User-controlled research means that decision-making power is with service users.

The concept of levels of involvement is important because it raises issues about decision-making power and the different types of knowledge that are valued and privileged in the research. Some authors have argued that there is a connection between higher levels of involvement and the empowerment of service users (Poulton 1999). Another way of describing this connection is 'tokenism' versus 'meaningful involvement'. However, involvement at different levels should not be judged as being better than another because it overlooks the fact that service user involvement has different purposes in different contexts. Some examples of the broad spectrum of activities associated with different levels of involvement are provided in Box 2.3.

Box 2.3   Levels of service user involvement

Consultation

- Surveys seeking general public opinions about health issues
- Participating in public opinion surveys about health services
- Patient surveys/satisfaction surveys
- Providing perceptions of participation in clinical/research trials

Contribution

- Conveying the patient/carer experience of health and illness as a lay member of a research team
- Direct involvement in research to inform service development or re-design
- Direct involvement in the design of trials/research questions, systematic reviews or scoping exercises
- Contributing to evaluations of clinical interventions, treatment or care giving practices
- Planned/strategic involvement of service users within research organisations, for example as part of a steering group or a service user reference group
- Service users involved in recruitment to research
- Involvement in the development and validation of research instruments or scales
- Service users involved in data collection, for example peer-interviewing
- Service users contribute to the analysis or interpretation of research data
- Service users contribute their views about the quality of their involvement in the research

Collaboration

- Co-applicant in proposal/protocol development for funding
- Partnership-based evaluation of health services
- Developing patient defined measures, tools or instruments
- Actively being involved in decisions about research agendas or priorities
- Direct involvement in commissioning/tendering or programme reviews
- Service users undertake the planned dissemination of research findings to service user audiences
- Service users as co-authors of research publications

Control

- Academic user researchers who lead on research studies
- User-controlled research
- Carer-controlled research
- Providing perspectives of the experience of service user involvement
- Service users use findings to influence commissioning or service change

---

A participation continuum

Service user involvement in decision-making has been related to notions of consumerist and democratic concepts of involvement (Hickey and Kipping 1998). These approaches are linked through a 'participation continuum', as illustrated by Figure 2.5. This arrangement challenges a hierarchical view of service user involvement as having levels of control, by suggesting that service user roles can exist simultaneously or merge into one another.

The idea of 'participation for purpose' is reconfirmed by concepts of deliberative participation internationally, for example a spectrum of levels of participation developed by the International Association for Public participation (Involve 2005). This model defines goals for public participation as follows:

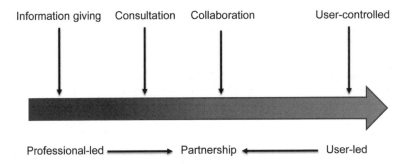

Figure 2.5 Participation as a continuum.

- *Inform* – To provide the public with balanced and objective information to assist them in understanding the problem, alternatives, opportunities and/or structures.
- *Consult* – To obtain public feedback on analysis, alternatives and/or decisions.
- *Involve* – To work directly with the public throughout the process to ensure that public concerns and aspirations are consistently understood and considered.
- *Collaborate* – To partner with the public in each aspect of the decision including the development of alternatives and the identification of the preferred solution.
- *Empower* – To place final decision-making in the hands of the public.

Overall there are limitations to existing models of service user involvement. The models tend to overlook broader aspects of service user involvement activities, such as involvement through ongoing collaborative relationships between research organisations and service user groups. Neither do they sufficiently reflect the contribution of service user involvement to international research collaborations, community–university partnerships, large-scale human/environmental health programmes and multidisciplinary research partnerships.

In the absence of more sophisticated models researchers within specific areas of health research are beginning to provide more detailed and critical accounts of service user involvement in research studies. For example, in a study by Grocott et al. (2007) on medical device development the relationship between service users, researchers and industry partners is made more explicit. Or, for example the work of Wilkinson et al. (2003) including people with dementia and their carers to promote partnership and prevent inappropriate hospital admissions. In another study from the USA (MacQueen and Cates 2005), a framework for prevention science clinical research has been devised (drawing on advocacy and policy, community participation, prevention research, acceptability research, and operations and programme development) to explicitly link service user need to the implementation of results in public health programmes.

A theoretical framework for approaching service user involvement in research

A helpful way of understanding service user involvement in research is to think of it as having four interrelated components (Smith et al. 2008). These are: context, methods, roles and outcomes. As illustrated by Figure 2.6, each of these components contains a

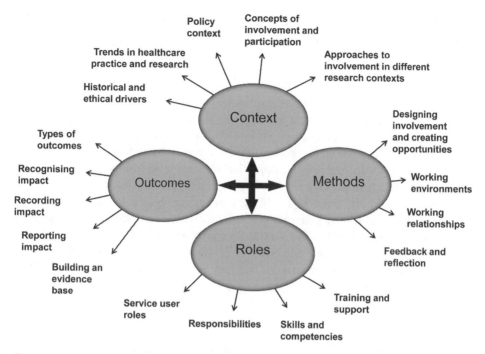

Figure 2.6   A framework of service user involvement in research.

cluster of issues and potential areas of learning. The four areas are summarised below and issues are cross referenced to parts of the book where further detail can be found.

Context

The context of service user involvement in nursing and healthcare research includes many of the issues discussed so far, such as the different meanings and ways of approaching service user involvement that we looked at in Chapter 1. Although we are focusing on research in this handbook, part of the context is being aware of parallel trends to involve service users in the commissioning, design and evaluation of health and social care research. As we also saw in Chapter 1, across many Westernised nations there is strong interest in engaging the public more actively in a wide-range of professional areas of working, including healthcare delivery, service design and health and social care research. The drivers for service user involvement include a range of historical and ethical reasons, including challenges to medical authority, changing roles of patients in policy, user-led research, democratisation of public services and public responses to professional scandals (Chapter 1). Part of the context of service user involvement in research is appreciating the different perspectives that people have towards it, and in particular how different approaches to service user involvement have developed in different research contexts (which we will look at in Chapter 3). As discussed in the first part of this chapter the terms of 'service user', 'carer' and 'involvement' are themselves open to interpretation and can be a cause of confusion. In this chapter we have also looked at how key concepts such as representation, experiential knowledge and meaningful involvement influence how service user involvement is thought of.

Methods

The second component of service user involvement in research is methods. As we will see in Chapter 3, designing involvement means giving attention to who to involve, building in opportunities for involvement, planning and costing involvement, and ensuring that requirements for research ethics and governance are met. Methods issues also include practical techniques for developing supportive working relationships, such as making connections, supportive working environments, defining roles and responsibilities, developing ways of working, being aware of legal and ethical issues, training and support, communication, and feedback and reflection. These issues are discussed in Chapter 4 along with the issue of embedding service user involvement within research organisations. Methods also include issues to be aware of when working with different groups of patients, clients and carers (Chapter 5), different age groups (Chapter 6) and seldom-heard groups (Chapter 7).

Roles

The third component of service user involvement in research is roles. It concerns the different types of research roles that service users might enter into, for example undertaking personal health research, joining a voluntary health network, service user-led organisation, charity or not-for-profit organisation, as well as becoming experienced service user representatives or academic service user-researchers (Chapter 8). It also concerns issues about researcher roles and the personal skills and capacity of researchers to involve service users in their work. For example, researchers can learn about indicators of successful involvement, how to document service user involvement work and how to make use of reflective techniques and reflexivity to build towards quality experiences of involvement and quality environments for involvement (Chapter 9).

Outcomes

The fourth component of service user involvement in research is outcomes. It includes issues about why we need to know about impact, the types of impact that may be expected, recognising, recording and reporting impact (Chapter 10).

Key principles for practice

- When talking and thinking about service user involvement in research be aware that the language is rapidly developing in this field and different terms are used to mean different things in different research and healthcare contexts. The terms 'service user' and 'carer' may be used to mean many different types of individuals, groups and organisations.

- Service user involvement in research concerns many interlinked concepts and ideas. Key concepts to be aware of are 'involvement', 'representation', 'experiential knowledge', 'participation' and 'empowerment'.
- Models of involvement can be useful for describing the intended approach. However, how service user involvement is played out is likely to change over time as researchers and service users become more aware of each other's strengths and contributions to the research.
- Service user involvement in research can be thought of as having four interrelated components: context, methods, roles and outcomes. These are each areas for personal and professional learning.

References

Arnstein, S. (1969) A ladder of citizen participation. *Journal of the American Institute of Planners*, 35 (4): 216–24.

Barnes, M. and Wistow, G. (1994) Achieving a strategy for user involvement in community care. *Health & Social Care in the Community*, 2: 347–56.

Beresford, P. (2003) *It's Our Lives: A Short Theory of Knowledge, Distance and Experience*. London: Citizen Press in association with Shaping Our Lives, pp. 1–59.

Beresford, P. (2005) 'Service user': regressive or liberatory terminology? *Disability & Society*, 20 (4): 469–77.

Beresford, P. (2007) User involvement, research and health inequalities: developing new directions. *Health & Social Care in the Community*, 15 (4): 306–12.

Beresford, P. and Campbell, J. (1994) Disabled people, service users, user involvement and representation. *Disability & Society*, 9 (3): 315–25.

Beresford, P. and Croft, S. (1996) The politics of participation. In: Taylor, D. (ed) *Critical Social Policy: A Reader*. London: Sage.

Bhavnani, K. (1990) What's power got to do with it? Empowerment and social research. In: Parker, I. and Shotter, J. (eds) *Deconstructing Social Psychology*. London: Routledge.

Brooks, F. (2006) Nursing and public participation in health: An ethnographic study of a patient council. *International Journal of Nursing Studies*, 45 (1): 3–13.

Cahill, J. (1996) Patient participation: a concept analysis. *Journal of Advanced Nursing*, 24: 561–71.

Cayton, H. (2002) Patient and public involvement. *Journal of Health Service Research Policy*, 9 (4): 193–4.

Christopoulos, A. and Rose, J. (2006) *MORI's Participation Unit—Peer Research*. Harrow: Ipsos MORI Participation Unit.

Clegg, S. (1989) *Frameworks of Power*. London: Sage.

Coulter, A. (1999) Paternalism or partnership? *British Medical Journal*, 319 (7212): 719–20.

Cullum, N. (2000) Users' guides to the nursing literature: an introduction. *Evidence Based Nursing*, 3 (3): 71–2.

Davies, C., Wetherell, M., and Barnett, E. (2006) *Citizens at the Centre: Deliberative Participation in Healthcare Decisions*. Bristol: Policy Press.

Edwards, C. (2000) Accessing the user's perspective. *Health & Social Care in the Community*, 8 (6): 417–24.

Edwards, C. and Titchen, A. (2003) Research into patients' perspectives: relevance and usefulness of phenomenological sociology. *Journal of Advanced Nursing*, 44 (5): 450–60.

Entwistle, V., Renfrew, M., Yearley, S., Forrester, J., and Lamont, T. (1998) Lay perspectives: advantages for health research. *British Medical Journal*, 316: 463–6.

Entwistle, V., Tritter, J., and Calan, M. (2002) Researching experiences of cancer: the importance of methodology. *European Journal of Cancer Care*, 11 (3): 232–7.

Glasby, J. and Beresford, P. (2006) Who knows best? Evidence-based practice and the service user contribution. *Critical Social Policy*, 26 (1): 268–84.

Glasby, J. and Littlechild, R. (2001) Inappropriate hospital admissions: patient participation in research. *British Journal of Nursing*, 10 (11): 738–41.

Grocott, P., Weir, H., and Bridgelal Ram, M. (2007) A model of user engagement in medical device development. *International Journal of Health Care Quality Assurance*, 20 (6): 484–93.

Hickey, G. and Kipping, C. (1998) Exploring the concept of user involvement in mental health through a participation continuum. *Journal of Clinical Nursing*, 7 (1): 83–8.

INVOLVE (2004) *Involving Consumers in Research and Development in the NHS. Briefing Notes for Researchers*, 2nd en. Eastleigh: INVOLVE. (Available from: www.invo.org.uk)

Involve (2005) *People & Participation, How to Put Citizens at the Heart of Decision Making.* London: Involve. (Available from: http://involving.org)

Lidz, C. and Appelbaum, P. (2002) The therapeutic misconception: problems and solutions. *Medical Care*, 40 (9): S55–63.

Lohan, M. and Coleman, C. (2005) Explaining the absence of the lay voice in sexual health through sociological theories of healthcare. *Social Theory & Health*, 3: 83–104.

MacQueen, K. and Cates, Jr. W. (2005) The multiple layers of prevention science research. *American Journal of Preventive Medicine*, 28 (5): 491–5.

Marshall, S., Crowe, T., Oades, L., Deane, F., and Kavanagh, D. (2007) A review of consumer involvement in evaluations of case management: consistency with a recovery paradigm. *Psychiatric Services*, 58 (3): 396–401.

Mercer, G. (2002) Emancipatory disability research. In: Barnes, C., Oliver, M., and Barton, L. (eds) *Disability Studies Today*. Cambridge: Policy Press.

Needham, C. (2003) *Citizen-Consumers: New Labour's Marketplace Democracy*. London: Catalyst Forum.

Poulton, B. (1999) User involvement in identifying health needs and shaping and evaluating services: is it being realised? *Journal of Advanced Nursing*, 30 (6): 1289–96.

Pawson, R., Boaz, A., Grayson, L., Long, A., and Barnes, C. (2003) *Types and Quality of Knowledge in Social Care. Knowledge Review 3*. London: Social Care Institute for Excellence. (Available from: www.scie.org.uk/publications/list.asp)

Popay, J. and Williams, G. (1998) Qualitative research and evidence-based healthcare. *Journal of the Royal Society of Medicine*, 191 (S35): 32–7.

Rhodes, P., Nocon, A., Wright, J., and Harrison, S. (2001) Involving patients in research. Setting up a service users' advisory group. *Journal of Management in Medicine*, 15 (2): 167–71.

Rodgers, J. (1994) If consumer involvement in health services is to be more than notional, users need to be empowered, not just consulted. *Health Service Journal*, 104: 28.

Rodwell, C. (1996) An analysis of the concept of empowerment. *Journal of Advanced Nursing*, 23 (2): 305–13.

Ross, F., Donovan, S., Brearley, S., Victor, C., Cottee, M., Crowther, P., and Clark, E. (2005) Involving older people in research: methodological issues. *Health & Social Care in the Community*, 13 (3): 268–75.

Rothwell, P.M. (2005) External validity of randomized controlled trials: to whom do the benefits apply? *Lancet*, 365: 82–93.

Russell, D., Hamilton, W., and Luthra, M. (2002) Research and consumer representation. *British Journal of General Practice*, 52 (474): 58.

Ryan, M., Scott, D., Bate, A., Napper, M., Robb, C., Reeves, C., van Teijlingen, E., and Russell, E. (2001) Eliciting public preferences for healthcare: a systematic review of techniques. *Health Technology Assessment*, 5 (5): 1–186.

Sackett, D., Rosenburg, W., Muir Gray, J.A., Haynes, R.B., and Richardson, S.W. (1996) Evidence-based medicine: what it is and what it isn't. *British Medical Journal*, 312: 71–2.

Seymour, J. and Skilbeck, J. (2002) Ethical considerations in researching user views. *European Journal of Cancer Care*, 11 (3): 215–9.

Smith, E., Ross, F., Donovan, S., Manthorpe, G., Brearley, S., Sitzia, J., and Beresford, P. (2008) Service user involvement in the design and undertaking of nursing, midwifery and health visiting research. *International Journal of Nursing Studies*, 45: 298–315.

Sweeney, A. and Morgan, L. (2009) The levels and stages of service user/survivor involvement in research. In: Wallcraft, J., Schrank, B., and Amering, M., (eds) *Handbook of Service User Involvement in Mental Health Research*. Chichester: Wiley-Blackwell.

Tritter, J. and McCallum, T. (2006) The snakes and ladders of user involvement. Moving beyond Arnstein. *Health Policy*, 76 (2): 156–68.

Turner, P. and Beresford, P. (2005) *User Controlled Research: Its Meanings and Potential. Final Report*. INVOLVE, Shaping Our Lives and the Centre for Citizen Participation, Brunel University. Eastleigh: INVOLVE.

Wilkinson, H., Bowes, A., and Rodrigues, A. (2003) Innovative methodologies – can we learn from including people with dementia from South Asian communities. *Research Policy & Planning*, 21 (2): 43–54.

Chapter 3

Designing involvement

Key summary points

- *Deciding who to involve*: Depending on the nature of the research different types of service users may be involved, such as people with direct experience of a health issue, people with direct experiences/opinions of health services, patient representatives, patient advocates, carers, community representatives, national service user representatives.
- *Building in opportunities for involvement*: Researchers should look for opportunities and avoid creating false expectations by considering involvement at different stages from designing, undertaking and evaluating the research. In most circumstances service users or carers can be involved in more than one type of activity as well as in decisions about planning and managing the research.
- *Research methods and approaches to involvement*: Some research studies aim to test an intervention, such as a treatment or procedure, and may use randomised or controlled methods. This type of study may follow an *experimental/clinical trials approach to involvement*. Other studies aim to elicit patient or staff perspectives of health issues. Such studies are more likely to follow a *qualitative approach to service user involvement*. Studies that involve the synthesis of previous research may follow a *systematic review approach* to service user involvement. Other research studies aim to directly bring about changes in patient care or to develop practice. These studies may use an *action research approach* to involve service users. In an *emancipatory approach* the research is controlled by users from the beginning of the process.
- *Planning involvement*: It can help to break down steps of involvement according to key aims and objectives, clarify the actions and time required and who will be responsible. Planning can also help to clarify expectations about what will happen and for service users who are involved to express their views about which aspects of the research they feel they can contribute to.
- *Costing and payments*: A participation fee should be offered that relates to the level of commitment required. Consideration should always be given to a person's wishes, impact on social security benefits and the method of payment. Always pay travelling expenses and carer costs. Try to pay expenses up-front or directly and keep financial records of payment.

Handbook of Service User Involvement in Nursing and Healthcare Research, First Edition.
Elizabeth Morrow, Annette Boaz, Sally Brearley and Fiona Ross.
© 2012 Elizabeth Morrow, Annette Boaz, Sally Brearley and Fiona Ross.
Published 2012 by Blackwell Publishing Ltd.

- *Research ethics and governance*: Different countries have different laws that govern nursing and healthcare research. Key issues researchers may need to be aware of are human and civil rights, when to seek formal ethical approval for service user involvement, the difference between ethical issues of research participation and the ethical issues of service user involvement in research.

Deciding who to involve

People with direct experience of a health issue

Some service users have in-depth personal experience of a medical condition or health issue, which can be useful for understanding issues that might be important for research to address. Involving such groups of service users means paying attention to personal factors, especially the severity of a person's illness, the length of time they have lived with a condition and their response to treatment. These issues are discussed further in Chapter 6. For ethical and practical reasons it is necessary to develop sensitive and flexible research methods which can accommodate service users who may not always be well enough to be involved in the research. Although numerous barriers and tensions have been identified to involving patients at a design stage, there is also evidence that patients can help to review consent procedures and patient information sheets, suggest outcomes for the research, review the acceptability of data collection procedures and make recommendations about the timing of approaches to participants (Boote et al. 2010).

People with direct experiences/opinions of health services

In studies about service evaluation, service users have been targeted because of their experience of accessing a particular health or social care service. In service development projects that aim to improve access to services, selected groups have been recruited because of demographics such as age or ethnic group. Researchers working to engage community members in public health research have reported that people are keen to be heard in the formulation of research but that competing demands and limited resources make it difficult for community groups to allocate scarce resources to consultation (Graham et al. 2001). Sometimes research issues may seem 'academic' and thus remote from the urgent priorities of the people with whom researchers wish to work.

Patient representatives

Involving patient representatives has been criticised for not being representative of all patients or all service users. Gaining the views or opinions that are representative of a group of service users can be achieved using research sampling and research methods (as previously discussed in Chapter 2). However these methods do not lend themselves easily to involving service users actively throughout decision-making processes because of the cost and time implications.

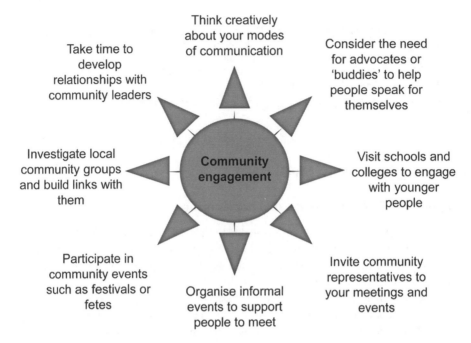

Take time to develop relationships with community leaders

Think creatively about your modes of communication

Consider the need for advocates or 'buddies' to help people speak for themselves

Investigate local community groups and build links with them

Community engagement

Visit schools and colleges to engage with younger people

Participate in community events such as festivals or fetes

Organise informal events to support people to meet

Invite community representatives to your meetings and events

Figure 3.1   Strategies for involving communities in research.

Patient advocates

Involving patient advocates, for example from statutory organisations or volunteer networks, can mean that a service user perspective is represented. This means that service users' stake in an issue is recognised and service user perspectives are included in the research. Trained patient advocates can provide insight into issues affecting patients and clinical practice, and are often able to ask pertinent questions because they recognise issues that professionals might overlook (Griffiths et al. 2003). However, when service users might have a high level of expertise and training, concern has been expressed that these people do not have close enough experience of patient issues.

Carers

Carers are not patients, though arguably they are users of services. Carers have a close knowledge of the person they care for, including their history and when something is wrong. But, they have a different perspective of the issues from the people they care for. Carers' views are important because researchers and clinicians may be focusing on symptoms at the expense of a more holistic day-to-day view of a person's needs or condition. The contribution of carers to research is discussed in more detail in Chapter 5.

Community representatives

Gaining access to under-researched groups is a particular challenge and requires specific planning (Berg 1999). Figure 3.1 illustrates some of the techniques utilised by researchers

---

Box 3.1   Factors supporting community involvement in research

Principles which can support community involvement:
- See the community as a unit of Identity
- Build on strengths and resources within the community
- Facilitate co-learning and co-construction of meaning
- Ensure community involvement in all stages
- See the process as cyclical and iterative
- Co-ownership of knowledge

Processes which can support community involvement:
- Time for collaboration
- Community participation at all stages
- Open access to key events

Structures which can support community involvement:
- Joint development of infrastructure
- Leadership from the community
- Community staffing and planning
- Collective access to resources/funding

Relationships which can support community involvement:
- Frequent and open communication
- Flexibility from all partners
- Awareness of historical influences

---

to engage communities, including obtaining the support and endorsement of community leaders and advertising the research in community publications.

Since each cultural group has unique issues and concerns, researchers must familiarise themselves with the values of their target group and emphasise these in recruitment approaches. A review of community-based participatory literature (Lencucha et al. 2010) shows that a number of factors can support community involvement, summarised in Box 3.1.

National service user representatives

Few studies have addressed representation of service user, carer and patients' interests nationally. Consumer and voluntary health groups have an important role in representing the collective interests of patients, service users and carers. A survey of consumer groups showed that the majority (80% of respondents) identified influencing policy at national level as 'very important' or 'important' (Jones et al. 2004). The survey showed that key facilitators in involving service users at a national level are:

- Recognition of experiential knowledge
- A clear agenda
- A transparent decision-making process
- Sufficient time
- Sufficient resources
- Established/ongoing working relationships with decision-makers
- Service users working in alliances with other health consumer groups or other stakeholders

Building in opportunities for involvement

Some people are of the view that service user involvement should be all the way through, at every stage, of a research study. However, this is often more an aspiration than a feasible way of working because of resource and time limitations. It can be a challenge for researchers to adopt new ways of working and to share the research process with patients and service user representatives, a point illustrated by the following case study (Box 3.2). Researchers may feel that service user involvement will take up too much time at proposal stage or raise expectations about the study being

---

Box 3.2   Working with research teams to develop service user involvement

Case study

Sophie Auckland, User Involvement Manager

I am the User Involvement Manager for Guy's and St. Thomas' Foundation Trust and King's College London Biomedical Research Centre. My role is to support researchers to implement service user involvement in the translational research activities of the Biomedical Research Centre. This means informing and advising academic and clinical research staff in a wide range of research areas including laboratory research, clinical trials and qualitative studies. The overall aim is that service user involvement will become a natural part of the research process.

'Starting out'

The competitive nature of research often motivates researchers to incorporate service user involvement into their applications for research funding. Some researchers want to know what benefits service user involvement will bring to their research before they attempt it – but to determine the benefits requires some service user involvement activity to take place in the first place. Part of my role is to collate examples of service user involvement and to work with academic researchers to assess its effectiveness. I encourage those researchers who have undertaken service user involvement to share their experiences and reflect on the impact it has had on their research. This information is scarce and more is needed to determine appropriate methods and the potential added value of service user involvement.

In the first instance many researchers need to know what service user involvement is and how to do it. To address this issue I have produced guidance to explain what distinguishes service user involvement from Public Engagement in Science, qualitative research methods and recruiting people to trials. Other common questions are how to recruit and retain service users for service user involvement and ways in which service user involvement can be implemented with real examples of how other researchers have put it into practice. As researchers work in different contexts and topic areas it is best to provide a range of support, such as written guidance, web materials or bespoke workshops with researchers and service users.

Key issues to be aware of:

• Some concerns and assumptions come up time and again. These are that service user involvement is time consuming and will delay the research, researchers are uncertain how much additional resources are required, whether it requires ethical approval and whether it will increase chances of being awarded funding.

- Service user involvement training for researchers can provide information and suggest alternatives to more traditional research processes. For example, suggesting a researcher go to a patient group meeting to discuss ideas is a much more efficient use of time and resources than setting up a service user group for one study.
- A challenge for researchers is to adopt new ways of working and to share the research process with patients and user representatives, and for service users to understand how they can contribute to the research. Both sides need to see the benefit to getting involved in a research partnership.

Helpful ideas:

- Researchers need to know about service user involvement – training and information is available.
- When starting out make service user involvement more manageable by identifying one or two stages of the research to begin with, for example developing the research design or tools.
- Experienced facilitators can help to create spaces where clinicians, academics and service users can communicate and discuss ideas together in a productive way.
- Research organisations can showcase local service user involvement activity and enable researchers to learn from one another, this can also help inform patients and the public about research and how they might be involved.

funded. For these reasons it is even more important to be clear about whether the research has been funded or not and what types of opportunities there could be for service user involvement. Where possible, seek support from experienced colleagues and work with service users in the early stages of planning a study to maximise opportunities for involvement.

Researchers should avoid creating false expectations about what is achievable by discussing involvement with service users at different stages of the research. Figure 3.2 is a typology of service user involvement activities that has been developed from a review of service user involvement in nursing, midwifery and health visiting research (Smith et al. 2008). The typology is helpful for considering different forms of service user involvement at different stages of *designing*, *undertaking* and *evaluating* research, whether in a one-off study on ongoing programme of work.

The following list (Table 3.1) provides greater detail of some of the range of roles and activities of service users that have been reported in the research literature at different stages of the research. These activities are often closely linked to the research method and the approach to involvement (discussed in the next section). In most studies service users or carers are involved in more than one type of activity as well as in decisions about planning and managing the research. As discussed in Chapter 2, researchers should be aware that some activities are perceived as relating to a low level of involvement (e.g. consultation) and others to a high level of involvement (e.g. the role of co-researcher).

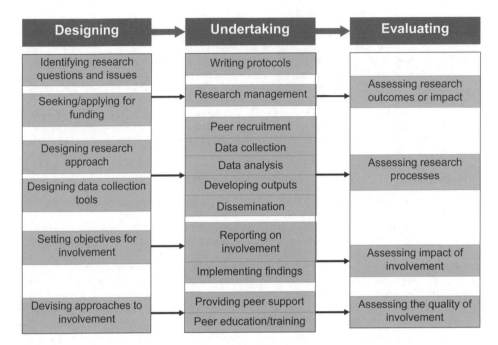

Figure 3.2   Typology of service user involvement in research.

Research methods and approaches to involvement

Service user involvement can help to support all types of nursing and healthcare research. Deciding upon which type of research methods to use is something that can be undertaken in partnership with service users. However, in most cases research commissioners and research teams will already have firm ideas about which types of methods will best address the questions at hand. Another factor in how service user involvement develops in a study is that different researchers will be more experienced and confident to use qualitative, quantitative or mixed-method approaches.

Nursing and healthcare research could make use of a wide range of approaches to collect and analyse different types of data, such as:

- Research papers and reports (e.g. systematic review)
- Clinical or non-clinical documents (e.g. patient notes or clinical protocols)
- Patient data (e.g. public health records or patient databases)
- Demographic/population data (e.g. health profiling or prevalence studies)
- Survey data (e.g. community health status or access to services)
- Observations (e.g. non-participant observation of treatments or procedures)
- Clinical measures (e.g. intervention studies)
- Quality of life outcomes (e.g. comparative studies)
- Personal accounts or experiences (e.g. focus groups or interviews)

Table 3.1 Service user roles and activities.

Designing	
Identifying research questions and issues	Identifying needs, problems or issues Developing new ideas for research Prioritising research questions
Seeking funding/applying for funding	Knowledge of potential funding sources Developing research proposals Submitting funding applications
Designing research approach	Choosing research approach (e.g. quantitative/qualitative) Knowledge of previous research findings and key concepts
Designing data collection tools	Contributing to questionnaire design Choosing suitable outcome measures Designing ways of capturing data, e.g. patient experiences
Setting objectives for involvement	Helping to identify stages of the research for involvement Writing terms of reference or objectives for involvement in the research Planning activities for service users to be involved in the research
Devising approaches to involvement	Involving community members Deciding the most appropriate times and places of involvement Helping to choose and create safe accessible environments for involvement
Undertaking	
Writing research protocols	Planning how the research will proceed Developing the aims and objectives of the research Writing lay summaries/leaflets about the planned research
Research management	Involvement in research ethics approval processes Contributing to research governance approval processes Costing the research or budgeting for involvement Managing personal research expenses/payments
Peer recruitment	Identifying target individuals or communities Talking to existing service user groups about participating in the research Providing potential participants with information about the research
Data collection	Administering questionnaires Undertaking interviews Co-facilitating focus groups

(*Continued*)

Table 3.1   (*cont'd*)

Data analysis	Identifying questions or issues for the analysis to address Naming or creating categories with which to analyse the data Choosing statistical tests to apply Providing a perspective on the categories chosen for use in an analysis Identifying issues or themes within the data Checking a researcher's application of categories to an interview
Developing outputs	Authorship of sections of the report Drafting or contributing to writing a paper Writing a case study
Disseminating the research	Co-presenting at conferences Attending public dissemination events and meetings Creating research posters Audio accounts (online stories) or radio broadcasts Digital/video presentations Web-based resources and information Designing newsletters/leaflets
Reporting on involvement	Keeping records of attendance/participation Keeping minutes of meetings Writing accounts of involvement activities
Providing peer support	Participating in 'buddy' systems Developing ground rules/best practices
Peer education/training	Attending training to carry out the research Shared learning events with research teams Contributing to training of other service users
Evaluating Assessing research outcomes or impact	Identifying types of impact, e.g. on patients, health systems or society
Assessing research processes	Evaluating processes of recruitment, data collection, analysis, development of outputs, dissemination, etc. Suggesting how processes could be improved
Assessing the impact of involvement	Identifying the types of contributions service users have made to the research Explaining how service users have influenced decisions made about the research
Assessing the quality of involvement	Evaluating how service users were involved in devising the approach to involvement in the research Evaluating peer support or education and training for service users who have been involved

Research studies tend to fall into four broad methodological categories:

- Some studies aim to test an intervention, such as a treatment or procedure, and may use randomised or controlled methods. This type of study may follow an *experimental/ clinical trials approach to involvement*.
- Other studies aim to elicit patient or staff perspectives of health issues. Such studies are more likely to follow a *qualitative approach to service user involvement*.
- Studies that purely involve the analysis of previous research may follow a *systematic review approach* to service user involvement.
- Other research will aim to bring about changes in patient care or to develop practice. These studies may use an *action research approach* to involve service users.

Experimental/clinical trials approach to involvement

Increasingly researchers leading clinical trials are making use of service user involvement to better understand the views and perceptions of research participants. This is helping to inform future recruitment practices, particularly in groups that are traditionally less likely to participate in trials, particularly ethnic minority groups. This type of research is generally classified as being quantitative because it involves using methods of randomisation, controlled samples to achieve statistically generaliseable findings. Increasingly, eliciting the views of potential participants is a necessary step in rigorous clinical trial development because consideration of patient preferences and motivations can ensure the best fit between interventions and goals (Rodeheaver et al. 2003). Increasingly service users are also being involved in the design of recruitment materials to trials or procedures for recruitment. Research has also been undertaken to gain an understanding of participants' experiences of being involved in a research trial, for example Dougherty et al. (1999) patient participation in a clinical trial of angina management, and Donovan et al. (2002) capture users' experiences of participating in cancer trials. Participating in clinical research trials has helped some patients with cancer to construct their lives meaningfully by providing a supportive structure and enabling a sense of hope (Moore 2001). This type of research is most often conducted as follow-up studies after a trial has completed, rather than at the time the person was a participant in the trial. Although this type of research has shown to be informative for the design and conduct of clinical trials this approach to involvement might be viewed as evaluative consultation (see models of involvement described in 'Representation' section of Chapter 2) rather than service user involvement in research because the researchers retain overall control of how service users' views are, or are not, used.

　Qualitative studies have also been used to inform trial management practices. In cancer treatment, Cox (2000) explored patients' views and experiences using in-depth interviews and quality of life questionnaires, at the beginning of, during and after trial participation. The findings provide insight and understanding in terms of the experience of trial involvement over time as well as the importance of meeting patients' information, decision-making and support needs. Cox (2000) recommends that managers of clinical trials focus on acknowledging the contribution trial participants make to cancer research, enhancing the process of preparing patients for trial participation, recognising the need for continuing care, the incorporation of patients and potential patients' views into the clinical trials system, and educating the public about clinical trials.

There is less evidence to show that service users have been involved in the design of research trials or in influencing the questions that the research sought to address. A national survey of service user involvement in designing, conducting and interpreting randomised controlled trials (Hanley et al. 2001) assessed the extent to which service users were involved in the work of 103 clinical trial coordinating centres in the UK. Responses from investigators about 48 individual trials were mostly positive, with respondents commenting that input from service users had helped refine research questions, improve the quality of patient information and make trials more relevant to the needs of patients. The authors conclude that service user involvement in the design and conduct of controlled trials seems to be growing, seems to be welcomed by most researchers, and seems likely to improve the relevance to users of the questions addressed and the results obtained.

Qualitative research approach to involvement

Qualitative research aims to gather an in-depth understanding of human behaviour and the reasons behind such behaviour. It can also include the study of human experiences and perceptions of an issue or phenomena, such as health or illness. Typically qualitative healthcare research uses smaller and more focused samples of patients or client groups than quantitative research. Researchers may spend considerable time interacting with such groups and opportunities to involve service users more actively in the research process may naturally arise. For example, qualitative researchers may use different approaches to collecting data, such as grounded theory, ethnography, phenomenology, or discourse analysis (Denzin and Lincoln 2005) and it can be useful to involve service users in verifying the types of interpretations and inferences that are made during the research. Service users can also be involved directly in determining which data are collected and how, such as interviews and group discussions, observation, reflective field notes and documentary sources. Qualitative analytic methods aim to take account of complexity, detail and context. Working with service users during the analysis can help to ensure that subtle differences in lay and professional language are not overlooked and that meaning is not misinterpreted (Cotterell 2008).

Systematic review approach to involvement

Although systematic reviews are increasingly being commissioned to inform policy development and provide recommendations for practice and research, when compared with other research contexts service user involvement is scarce and highly variable (Braye and Preston-Shoot 2005). Methods of systematic review range from medical models, where statistics about effectiveness are amalgamated across several research trials, to qualitative approaches where information is gathered and synthesised to explore the scope of a topic or build an interpretation of the issues (Murphy et al. 1998; Petticrew and Roberts 2005), including approaches described as meta-analysis, systematic research synthesis, narrative review and realistic synthesis (Reason 2002); and classified as effectiveness-based, problem-based or theory based-approaches (Pawson and Boaz 2004). Some approaches align with qualitative research methods, including grounded theory, hermeneutics, and phenomenology; policy discourse analysis; or historical approaches to documentary analysis.

In the context of mental health research, Salvi et al. (2005) identify 35 systematic review studies that have involved service users. Of these, three studies were user-led. In three other studies the users were simply consulted but did not have any active role in the research. The remaining 29 studies were based on collaboration between service users and professional researchers.

A review of the work of the Cochrane Collaboration (Gheresi 2002) reveals that different approaches to involvement have been tried and different levels of success have been achieved. Some Cochrane Review Groups have embraced the concept and been fortunate in their ability to identify willing and able contributors, such as the Consumer and Communication Review group (Kelson 1999). For other researchers, the main point of contention is awarding status to subjective experience in the process of compiling evidence (Glasby and Beresford 2006). There are also issues about when and how to incorporate lay knowledge into a tightly defined systematic process.

Action research approach to involvement

Action research methods focus on generating evidence with communities of people to bring about change. It is a participative process because community members decide what the main issues are and how best to go about collecting evidence for change. In this research context a 'community of practice' is not necessarily a geographically based social group. It could mean a group of patients who share a similar health condition, or healthcare staff working to develop practice in a particular clinical area. The key idea is that the community share a common interest in making change happen. Action research has close links with community development and health improvement. It engages the community in finding solutions to the problems or issues that are important to them through the Action Research Cycle (Lewin 1946). Essentially, researchers and community members work together through a spiral of steps to reflect, act, plan and observe. Different forms of action research have been developed, including Participative Action Research, Co-operative Inquiry, and Action Research in Organisational Development (Reason and Bradbury 2001).

In terms of service user involvement, in action research service users are most likely to be part of the community that is engaged in the research. However they may have a slightly different role than the main community members involved in the research, such as providing information to researchers about the best way to access communities in the first instance or explaining what type of issues may be important to them.

Emancipatory approaches

The term emancipation has been described as 'setting people free from the coercive constraint of more powerful or dominant other people or social groups' (Williamson 2010). In the context of nursing and healthcare research, emancipatory research is controlled by service users from the beginning of the process. It may also be defined as 'user-controlled' or 'user-led' research, though there are ideological differences in the underlying meaning of these terms (Beresford 2009). To date, most emancipatory research has made use of qualitative methods and feminist approaches to critique and explore societal norms of gender, race, class, sexuality and other social inequalities. However, this type of research is not about methods, it is about who has control. Any research method could potentially be adopted by a user-led group and used for emancipatory research. In a series of seminars across the UK (Hanley 2005), participants discussed issues about emancipatory approaches. A consensus emerged between the seminar participants that:

- Definitions of emancipatory research and service user involvement in research need to be debated and shared more widely.
- There is a need to evaluate best practice in emancipatory research.
- More funding is needed for emancipatory approaches. A proportion of funding being set aside for more emancipatory approaches would help to address some of the power imbalances.
- Emancipatory research needs to be judged by the same standards on involvement and purpose. The outcomes of the research in strengthening the community involved in the research are crucial.
- User-researchers have the same responsibilities to involve service users as conventional researchers, and emancipatory research cannot be an end in itself. For it to be valued by users it needs to lead to changes.

Planning involvement

Whichever research method or approach to involvement is being used service user involvement in research requires planning. Planning helps to make sure there is sufficient time set aside to work with service users rather than the process feeling rushed and haphazard. It can help to break down steps of involvement according to key aims and objectives. This approach helps to clarify the actions and time required and who will be responsible, as is illustrated by Figure 3.3. Planning can also help to clarify expectations about what will happen and for service users who are involved to express their views about which aspects of the research they feel they can contribute to.

Payments

Costing

In 2006, the UK government published 'Reward and Recognition' (Department of Health 2006), an important landmark document concerning reimbursement and payment for members of the public who contribute to health and social care services and research. This national guidance sets out a framework for the reimbursement of expenses and

Aims	Objectives	Actions required	Time required	Responsible persons	Monitoring and assessment	Links to other work
e.g. Recruit service user group for research project	Setting up and supporting a service user group	Link with community groups Promote study and involvement	2–3 months	Lead researcher with support from project advisory group	Membership, meetings, nature of input into project	Other service user groups in institution, link to project advisory group
e.g. Meet training and support needs of service users involved	Understand and address training and support needs of service users	Ask service users about their needs Seek guidance and support	3–4 weeks	Lead researcher with service users	Training preferences and uptake	External support groups, facilitation, project team support
e.g. Feedback to service users involved in the research	Inform and acknowledge contributions of service users to the research	Communication of main achievements by service user's preferred method	1–2 weeks (at three intervals in project)	Lead researcher with chair of service user group	Newsletters and feedback	Publications department Dissemination strategy

Figure 3.3   Key ideas for planning involvement.

payment of fees to service users involved in any aspect of research. When designing research it is important to budget adequately for service user involvement on the basis of how many people will be involved, the nature of their involvement and the duration of their involvement. Researchers should be aware that it can be both necessary and beneficial to negotiate issues such as rates of payment, conditions, and 'job descriptions' with local or national service user groups before a study starts. It is also important to be able to make clear from the outset *when* and *what* payment can be expected (see case study, Box 3.3), as this informs people's choices about whether or not to get involved.

There are likely to be additional 'indirect' costs associated with service user involvement. The research can take longer than it might otherwise – for example, extra time for recruitment, training and involvement in research tasks. Researchers need to outline the cost implications of involvement at proposal stage as well as identifying the related benefits of service user involvement. This includes providing details of proper support and training and any special provision that will be made to involve different types of service users in the research, for example, language translators. Key ideas for paying service users are summarised by Figure 3.4.

Whereas the costs of actively involving people who use services and members of the public can be built into applications for research funding, researchers may have already incurred expenditure for involvement before funding is given, for example, the costs of involving service users in writing a research proposal. At the present time, it is unlikely that these 'up-front' costs will be covered by research commissioners, but some are willing to fund pilot studies where service user involvement can be initiated and developed prior to embarking on a larger study.

Box 3.3   Older service users' views about payment

Case study

Sheila Donovan, Faculty of Health and Social Care Sciences, Kingston University and St George's, University of London

The first research project I worked on, a qualitative study about the risk of falls, had a consumer panel of older people working alongside the research team as part of its partnership approach (1). The team had no preconceived ideas or blueprint for how 'service user involvement' would work, or what it would look like in practice. Instead, we relied on our commitment to working with service users in this new way, and our openness with them about the project being an endeavour in which we would learn together. The ensuing learning has continued to inform my approach to research and my research practice ever since.

Paying members of a service user group

In 2005, a colleague and I set up and supported a service user group to offer guidance and advice on our respective research projects. The projects were led by the same principal investigator and set in the same locality, and they both focused on older people and falls prevention; one was about older people's participation in community exercise classes and the other was about the quality of care for older people who have fallen. Each project had an integral 'service user involvement' component and had been awarded funds from the research commissioners (a primary care trust and a charitable foundation respectively) to support this. In line with guidelines from INVOLVE (www.invo.org.uk), the plan was to reimburse individuals for any expenses they incurred, and to pay them for their time and expertise.

   Once the project had started we discovered that the service users we worked with had strong and disparate views about payment. The issue of payment was discussed over the course of three meetings and generated quite heated debate. The discussions even continued outside of scheduled meetings, between the service users themselves, and also between service users and researchers, in telephone conversations and, in one instance, through written correspondence initiated by a service user. One member was concerned that accepting money in this way might divert funds from the National Health Service. This person was not convinced by our explanations that research budgets were separate from funding for patient services, and expressed what seemed to be a fundamental disagreement with the whole idea of payment for service users. Others suggested that as the group's members were retired and had access to free public transport, there were no 'expenses' to be reimbursed. The opposite view was put forward that *not* paying service users could be a disincentive for some people. One member, who although no longer attending meetings, nevertheless completed an evaluation form we had distributed, highlighted the anomaly that the payment rate for attending research project meetings was significantly more than that offered for providing care for a relative.

Key issues to be aware of:

- Managing the issue of payment for service user involvement may mean more than simply adopting national and/or local guidelines. Payment can be an emotive issue and will require time and sensitivity.
- Administrative procedures within a project's host institution can be convoluted and service user-unfriendly. Find out early on about the requirements and time involved for processing payments for service users.
- Be clear about the rationale for service user involvement within an individual project. Our discussions about payment led to other conversations, including one about the value of service user involvement and the impact service users can have on a research study.

Helpful ideas:

- Allow service users to exercise choice. The service user group agreed that a practical solution was for individual members to either accept, decline or donate their payment to a health charity.
- Balance group discussions with one-to-one conversations. Payment is a personal and sensitive issue that should be discussed with individuals in confidence.
- Agree ground rules for the service user group at the outset and elect a confident and skilled chairperson. These can prove particularly invaluable when a group discusses sensitive issues.

(1) Ross, F., Donovan, S., Brearley, S., Victor, C., Cottee, M., Crowther, P., and Clark, E. (2005) Involving older people in research: methodological issues. *Health & Social Care in the Community*, 13 (3): 268–75.

➤ **Refer to available guidance** (e.g. Department of Health, Reward and Recognition 2006)
➤ **Budget for service user involvement**
➤ **Keep financial records**
➤ **Expenses:** Always pay travelling expenses (ask people to bring you their receipts). Always pay carer costs (e.g. personal assistance, child care). Try to pay expenses up-front or directly e.g. arranging and paying for taxis when needed, sending people parking tokens before meetings
➤ **Participation fees:** A fee should be offered that relates to the level of commitment required. Service users may want the fee to be paid to themselves, their organisations, a charity, or may not wish to receive a payment – this should be discussed with each person privately. Payments for children and young people should be given special consideration.
➤ **Payments may affect service user's social security benefits**: Encourage service users to seek appropriate advice
➤ **Ask service users how they prefer to be paid**: Some people may not have bank accounts or may prefer to receive vouchers rather than cash (but for tax reasons these will still count as income)
➤ **Assure payment is made promptly** or be clear when payment can be expected

Figure 3.4 Key ideas about payment.

Reimbursement of expenses

People who are involved in research should not end up financially worse off for participating, particularly as they are generally already making a significant personal contribution to the research. Reimbursement helps to ensure equal opportunities for participation. All out of pocket expenses should be reimbursed, including:

- Travel (public transport, taxi fares, or an agreed private car mileage rate which includes wear and tear)
- Overnight accommodation
- Subsistence (food and drinks bought whilst 'on business')
- Childcare
- Telephone/internet and access/fax costs
- Stationery/equipment
- Carer costs
- Costs of a Personal Assistant of the individual's choice
- Conference fees
- Participation in training

Always remind people to bring their receipts or tickets with them so that these can be reimbursed promptly. Where possible pay expenses up-front or directly, such as arranging and paying for taxis when needed, and sending people parking tokens before meetings.

Participation fees

There are a number of reasons for paying service users a participation fee. These include:

- Financially recognising the added value to research
- Creating an incentive for active involvement
- Helping to redress lay/professional imbalances
- Supporting inclusion by addressing financial constraints and implications of involvement
- Helping to clarify the level of responsibility relating to a person's involvement

A participation fee should be offered that relates to the level of commitment required. Rates paid will depend on a number of factors such as the:

- Level of skill, expertise, and experience required/being contributed
- Time commitments involved (including preparation, reading, travel, communication, meeting attendance)
- Comparative levels of pay and responsibility of other team members
- Level of responsibility and commitment expected
- Relative local and national pay conditions, such as national minimum wage
- Volunteer payment rates for equivalent roles

When offering payment it is essential to recognise that not all service users want the same thing. Some service users may want the fee to be paid to themselves, their organisations or a charity of their choice. This should be discussed with each individual in confidence to avoid a pressure to do what others are doing or to be seen to be doing the right thing. Some people might choose not to be paid because of altruism, financial circumstances, or because of the potential impact on social security benefits or tax. These are matters of individual choice and not reasons for avoiding the offer of payment in the first place. Payments might affect service users' social security benefits. This should be made known to individual service users so they can seek advice before deciding to become involved or to receive payment. People in receipt of state benefits and allowances have an obligation to declare changes in their circumstances. It is necessary to assure that financial records are kept for auditing and tax purposes.

Payments for children and young people raise different types of issues. Ethical concerns over payment for children's research participation tend to regard all forms of payment as equally suspect. However, payments to reimburse out-of-pocket expenses and to compensate for research time and burdens are ethically justifiable and should be paid. Small incentive payments or rewards may be acceptable when needed to ensure sufficient enrolment in important research. Giving small gifts as a 'thank you', as well as some supplies to local schools or youth organisations is a way of giving both individual and collective compensation for involvement.

Ask all service users how they prefer to be paid; some people may not have bank accounts or may prefer to receive vouchers rather than cash (but for tax reasons these will still count as income). Try to assure payment is made promptly and that service users are informed when payment can be expected.

Legal requirements

In the UK and most other Westernised countries, Employment Law applies wherever a person is being paid for a service. If you work in an organisation, the Human Resources department staff should be able to advise you about Employment Law.

For tax purposes:

- Reimbursement of expenses is generally not counted as income.
- Where members of the public are working in partnership with a research organisation, payments can often be arranged through the organisation's payroll system where any deductions can be made at source.
- Lump sum payments can be made to members of the public as 'contractors' or 'consultants' who are responsible for their self-assessed tax payments.
- If the member of public is part of an organisation or group which is being paid for consultancy work by a research organisation, then it may be possible for the organisation to deduct tax through its own payroll arrangements.

Non-financial rewards

Whether or not service users are awarded payments it is important to provide non-financial rewards for their involvement. Specifically, thanking and acknowledging individuals for their time and contributions helps to secure commitment and a sense of recognition. Benefiting from good working relationships can be as important as receiving payment. It is important to support service users in ways which enhance their capacity to contribute, for example, helping with literacy or access to information. Other types of personal benefits for individuals who get involved should also be discussed. These might include training and learning, attending conferences, confidence building, help with career development and gaining future employment.

Research ethics and governance

Different countries have different laws that govern nursing and healthcare research. Key issues researchers may need to be aware of are:

- Human and civil rights
- When to seek formal ethical approval for service user involvement
- The difference between ethical issues of research participation and ethical issues of service user involvement in research

---

Box 3.4   Human and civil rights relevant to service user involvement in research

Human rights

Universal Declaration of Human Rights was adopted by the United Nations General Assembly in 1948, partly in response to the atrocities of World War II. Although the UDHR was a non-binding resolution, it is now considered to have acquired the force of international customary law which may be invoked under appropriate circumstances by national and other judiciaries. The UDHR urges member nations to promote a number of human, civil, economic and social rights, asserting these rights are part of the 'foundation of freedom, justice and peace in the world.'

The three principal regional human rights instruments are the *African Charter on Human and Peoples' Rights*, the *American Convention on Human Rights* and the *European Convention on Human Rights*.

The United Nations treaties make rights binding on all states that have signed this treaty, creating human rights law. The seven core treaties are:

- Convention on the Elimination of All Forms of Racial Discrimination
- Convention on the Elimination of All Forms of Discrimination Against Women
- United Nations Convention Against Torture
- Convention on the Rights of the Child
- Convention on the Rights of Persons with Disabilities
- International Convention on the Protection of the Rights of All Migrant Workers and Members of their Families

Civil rights

Civil and political rights were among the first to be recognised and codified. In many countries, civil rights or 'constitutional' rights are included in a bill of rights or similar document. Civil and political rights need not be codified to be protected, although most democracies worldwide do have formal written guarantees of civil and political rights. Custom also plays a role even though not expressly guaranteed by written law. One example is the right to privacy. In many countries, citizens have greater protections against infringement of rights than non-citizens.

At a fundamental level anyone who participates in research has basic human and civil rights (Box 3.4). These rights guard against unjust suffering and discrimination. Individuals, including young people and children, have a right to have a say in matters that concern them.

Researchers and service users' responsibilities for research governance differ between research contexts. For this reason it is important to seek advice from research ethics committees or those with expertise in service user involvement to determine what the main ethical issues are in relation to any particular study. A statement has been developed by the National Research Ethics Service (NRES) and INVOLVE to provide clarity and guidance on patient and public involvement in research and the requirements of research ethics review (Box 3.5). The statement has been approved by the NRES Advisory Group on NHS Service Users and Ethical Review.

Box 3.5   Summary of NRES/INVOLVE agreement for ethical approval

Active involvement versus participation in research

Involvement in research as a research participant comes with the protection afforded by research governance arrangements that include research ethics committee (REC) review to protect the rights, safety, dignity and well-being of research participants.

However, when we talk about 'involvement' in research, in this statement, we mean getting actively involved in the research process itself, rather than being participants or subjects of the research. Many people describe public involvement in research as research that is done with or by the public, and not to, about, or for them. The public has been involved in research and development for a number of years and in a variety of different ways.

For example this includes:

• Identifying and prioritising research topics
• Being part of research advisory groups and steering groups
• Undertaking research projects
• Reporting and communicating research findings

When is ethical approval required for active involvement?

The active involvement of patients or members of the public does not generally raise any ethical concerns for the people who are actively involved, even when those people are recruited for this role via the NHS. This is because they are not acting in the same way as research participants. They are acting as specialist advisers, providing valuable knowledge and expertise based on their experience of a health condition or public health concern.

Therefore ethical approval is not needed for the active involvement element of the research (even when people are recruited via the NHS), where people are involved in planning or advising on research, for example helping to develop a protocol, questionnaire or information sheet, member of advisory group, or co-applicant.

Research requires ethical approval as determined by the Governance Arrangements for Research Ethics Committees (GAfREC) and legislation including the Clinical Trials Directive and Mental Capacity Act. The NRES website provides guidance on the requirements for ethical review (www.nres.npsa.nhs.uk). The ethics committee will not need to consider within its review the active involvement of patients and members of the public in carrying out research that involves no direct contact with study participants, for example helping to analyse survey data, postal surveys, etc. However, where people's involvement results in direct contact with study participants the ethics committee will need to give specific consideration to the involvement as an element of the ethical consideration and approval.

A REC will need to check that the person carrying out the research has adequate training, support and supervision appropriate to the circumstances in the usual way. Here there are two ethical issues to consider in addition to the usual concerns about the safety of researchers and the researcher/participant relationship:

- The well-being and safety of the people who are actively involved as researchers. They may find that talking to other people reminds them of their own negative experiences. This can cause distress, in which case the patient/member of the public who is carrying out the research may need additional counselling/support. A REC will need to check this additional support is available.
- The well-being and safety of the people who are taking part in the research as study participants. It is important to ensure that there are no additional risks to people taking part in a study. The REC will also need to consider any additional issues or sensitivities that may arise for those taking part in the research.

Key principles for practice

- Be clear about who is being involved – people with direct experience of a health issue, people with direct experiences/opinions of health services, patient representatives, patient advocates, carers, community representatives or national service user representatives.
- Consider different types of service user involvement at different stages of *designing*, *undertaking* and *evaluating* the research. Seek feedback from service users about how they think they might best contribute.
- Be aware that different approaches to service user involvement may be used within different research traditions and methods.
- Break down steps of involvement according to key aims and objectives, clarify the actions and time required and who will be responsible.
- Offer a participation fee that relates to the level of commitment required. Consider each person's wishes, impact on social security benefits and the method of payment. Always pay travelling expenses and carer costs. Try to pay expenses up-front or directly and keep financial records of payment.
- Be aware of research governance issues, human and civil rights, when to seek formal ethical approval for service user involvement, the difference between ethical issues of research participation and the ethical issues of service user involvement in research.

References

Beresford, P. (2009) User-controlled research. In: Wallcraft, J., Schrank, B., and Amering, M. (eds) *Handbook of Service User Involvement in Mental Health Research.* Chichester: Wiley-Blackwell.

Berg, J. (1999) Gaining access to under researched populations in women's health research. *Health Care for Women International,* 20 (3): 237–43.

Boote, J., Baird, W., and Beecroft, C. (2010) Public involvement at the design stage of primary health research: a narrative review of case examples. *Health Policy*, 95 (1): 10–23.

Braye, S. and Preston-Shoot, M. (2005) Emerging from out of the shadows? Service user involvement in systematic reviews. *Evidence & Policy*, 1 (2): 173–93.

Cotterell, P. (2008) Exploring the value of service user involvement in data analysis: 'Our interpretation is about what lies below the surface'. *Educational Action Research*, 16 (1): 5–17.

Cox, K. (2000) Enhancing cancer clinical trial management: recommendations from a qualitative study of trial participants' experiences. *Psycho-Oncology*, 9 (4): 314–22.

Denzin, N.K. and Lincoln, Y.S. (eds) (2005). *The Sage Handbook of Qualitative Research*, 3rd edn. Thousand Oaks, CA: Sage.

Department of Health (2006) *Reward and Recognition*. London: DH.

Donovan, J., Brindle, L., and Mills, N. (2002) Capturing users' experiences of participating in cancer trials. *European Journal of Cancer Care*, 11 (3): 210–4.

Dougherty, C., Nichol, W., Dewhurst, T., and Spertus, J. (1999) Patient perspectives on participation in a clinical trial of angina management. *Applied Nursing Research*, 12 (2): 107–11.

Ghersi D. (2002) Making it happen: approaches to involving consumers in Cochrane reviews. *Evaluation & the Health Professions*, 25 (3): 270–83.

Glasby J. and Beresford P. (2006) Who knows best? Evidence-based practice and the service user contribution. *Critical Social Policy*, 26 (1): 268–84.

Graham, J., Broom, D., and Whittaker, A. (2001) Consulting about consulting: challenges to effective consulting about public health research. *Health Expectations*, 4 (4): 209–12.

Griffiths, K., Jorm, A., and Christensen, H. (2003) Academic consumer researchers: a bridge between consumers and researchers. *Australian & New Zealand Journal of Psychiatry*, 38 (4): 191–6.

Hanley, B. (2005) User involvement in research: building on experience and developing standards. York, U.K.: Joseph Rowntree Foundation.

Hanley, B., Truesdale, A., King, A., Elbourne, D., and Chalmers, I. (2001) Involving consumers in designing, conducting, and interpreting randomised controlled trials: questionnaire survey. *British Medical Journal*, 322: 519–23.

Jones, K., Baggott, R., and Allsop, J. (2004) Influencing the national policy process: the role of health consumer groups. *Health Expectations*, 7(1): 18–28.

Kelson, M. (1999) Consumer collaboration, patient-defined outcomes and the preparation of Cochrane Reviews. *Health Expectations*, 2 (2): 129–35.

Lencucha, R., Kothari, A., and Hamel, N. (2010) Extending collaborations for knowledge translation: lessons from the community-based participatory research literature. *Evidence & Policy*, 6 (1): 61–75.

Lewin, K. (1946) Action research and minority problems. *Journal of Social Issues*, 2 (4): 34–46.

Moore, S. (2001) A need to try everything: patient participation in phase I trials. *Journal of Advanced Nursing*, 33 (6): 738–47.

Murphy, E., Dingwal, R., Greatbatch, D., Parker, S., and Watson, P. (1998) Qualitative research methods in health technology assessment: a review of the literature, Vol. 2, No. 16. London: Health Technology Assessment.

Pawson, R. and Boaz, A. (2004) Evidence-based policy, theory-based synthesis, user-led review: an ESRC Research Methods Programme Project. London: ESRC UK Centre for Evidence Based Policy and Practice.

Petticrew, M. and Roberts, H. (2005) *Systematic Reviews in the Social Sciences: A Practical Guide*. Oxford: Blackwell.

Reason, P. (2002) Evidence based policy: the promise of realist synthesis. *Evaluation*, 8 (3): 340–58.

Reason, P. and Bradbury, H. (eds) (2001) *Handbook of Action Research*. London: Sage.

Rodeheaver, P.F., Taylor, A.G., and Lyon, D.E. (2003) Incorporating patients' perspectives in complementary and alternative medicine clinical trial design. *Journal of Alternative & Complementary Medicine*, 9 (6): 959–67.

Salvi, G., Jones, J., and Ruggeri, M. (2005) Systematic review of the role of service users as researchers in mental health studies. *Epidemiologia e Psichiatria Sociale*, 14 (4): 217–26.

Smith, E., Ross, F., Donovan, S., Manthorpe, J., Brearley, S., Sitzia, J., and Beresford, P. (2008) Service user involvement in nursing, midwifery and health visiting research: a review of evidence and practice. *International Journal of Nursing Studies*, 45 (2): 298–315.

Williamson, C. (2010) *Towards the Emancipation of Patients. Patients' Experiences and the Patient Movement*. Bristol: The Policy Press.

Chapter 4

Working relationships

Key summary points

- *Making connections*: Researchers can connect with service users in a range of ways including through existing research relationships, clinical relationships, contact through local services, public advertisements, approaches to service user organisations and community groups. There should be a clear rationale for who is being approached and concise information should be provided about the purpose of the research and opportunities for involvement. Any personal information provided by service users should be held in confidence.
- *Working environments*: Research institutions or clinical environments may not always be the best place to develop good working relationships with service users. It can be beneficial to consult service users about the type of locations and working environments that are acceptable to them. Access is not only about access to buildings it is about providing people with equal opportunity to participate fully in the research by helping them to feel they are able to understand, communicate and participate in a way that suits them. Developing ground rules with service users helps to establish a preferred way of working and mutual respect.
- *Roles and responsibilities*: The types of responsibilities that service users involved in the research will have should be made clear so that these can be discussed and agreed as early on as possible. It can be useful to develop a 'job description' to define what a service user's role is in the research.
- *Legal and ethical issues*: Depending on the nature of the research and the type of service user involvement different legal and ethical issues will apply. In most situations it will be necessary for researchers to discuss general principles of confidentiality, data protection and informed consent with service users who are participating in the research.
- *Training and support*: It is good practice to offer service users training as part of being involved in the research. Training can vary in duration and formality from one-off interactive sessions with the research team to registering with an academic institution for personal study towards a research qualification.
- *Communication*: Communication is essential for developing good working relationships, engaging people in the research, promoting the research aims and objectives, and disseminating findings. Communication should be thought of as a two-way process that

---

Handbook of Service User Involvement in Nursing and Healthcare Research, First Edition.
Elizabeth Morrow, Annette Boaz, Sally Brearley and Fiona Ross.
© 2012 Elizabeth Morrow, Annette Boaz, Sally Brearley and Fiona Ross.
Published 2012 by Blackwell Publishing Ltd.

can follow a number of channels, including between members of the research team and service users, to wider stakeholders in the research, and to research, practice and service user audiences.

- *Feedback and reflection*: Feedback from the research team to service users who are involved is important for keeping people informed about how things are progressing and whether any changes in the research or involvement may need to be made. Feedback from service users to researchers can be used to make sure that involvement is working well. Reflective diaries, interviews, group discussions, feedback forms, suggestion boxes or reflection boards can be used to capture views and experiences.
- *Embedding service user involvement*: There are many advantages to developing service user involvement in research organisations. It can help to spread learning across whole programmes or research organisations, build expertise and develop best practice for ways of working and support systems.

Making connections

As discussed in Chapter 3, depending on the nature of the research different types of service users may be involved, such as people with direct experience of a health issue, people with direct experiences/opinions of health services, patient representatives, patient advocates, carers, community representatives and national service user representatives. Ways of making connections with service users are similarly diverse and can include:

- Through existing research relationships, for example, inviting participants in clinical trials to take a more active role in the research.
- Through existing clinical relationships, for example inviting people who attend a post-natal clinic to participate in a research project about how to improve the service.
- Promotion in local services, for example putting newsletters or posters in places where service users are likely to see them.
- Public advertisements, for example radio or articles in the press.
- Approaching service user organisations and networks, for example formally writing to invite (selected or elected) members to participate in the research.
- Approaching organisations, for example schools, local clubs and societies, and faith groups.
- Approaching community groups, for example speaking to a representative of a travelling community.

Preparation helps to get service user involvement off to a good start. Researchers will be familiar with processes of recruitment of participants to research studies, and to some extent making connections with service users is a similar process. General good practice is that:

- There should be a clear rationale for who is being approached, for example a recruitment framework identifying the types of service users that will be invited to be involved.

- Concise information (written if possible) should be provided about the purpose of the research, who is leading the work, timescales, funding source, etc.
- Information (written if possible) should be provided about possible opportunities for involvement, roles and responsibilities, and payment.
- Any personal information provided by service users to the research team, such as contact details, should be respected and maintained confidentially.
- It is useful to keep a log of responses (date, name, reason for enquiry, response given, etc.) to ensure details are not forgotten or lost, particularly if more than one research is working to make connections with service users.

Later in this chapter we will see that service users can take on different roles in the research, for example as co-researchers within the research team, as advisors to the research or as stakeholders. A popular way of engaging service users in research is inviting individuals to become members of a service user reference or advisory group specifically to work on a research study or programme. Service user groups are advantageous because multiple service users are involved and can bring different service user perspectives to the research. Researchers from the north of England who set up a service users' advisory group as part of a diabetes service evaluation recommend that a precise role for the group should be specified at the outset, that genuine service user involvement is needed, wide and accurate representation of all relevant groups in society is essential, and that researchers must approach service users with open minds with a view to shared decision-making rather than control (Rhodes et al. 2001). Factors that contributed to the group's success included personal contact, continuity of membership and integration into the management structure of the project. Also valued were the confidence in numbers which membership of the group gave, and the opportunity to meet and discuss issues away from the formal and somewhat intimidating atmosphere of the project's steering group. Aside from the personal value to participants and any impact on the quality of research outcomes, wider benefits included the ability to share knowledge with others and gain greater intercultural understanding (Rhodes et al. 2002). Service user groups can take time to set up and for good working relationships to evolve. Groups need to be supported, either by researchers or an appointed service user who acts as a chairperson. The size of a group will vary depending on the nature of the research, the model of involvement and the resources that are available for involvement. Figure 4.1 summarises some key ideas for establishing an effective service user group.

Working environments

There can be barriers or challenges to connecting with service users. These are sometimes referred to as access issues. Access is not only about access to buildings, it is about providing people with equal opportunity to participate fully in the research. Every individual person has different access needs – access is about helping people feel they are able to understand, communicate and participate in a way that suits them. Figure 4.2

> ➤ **Establish some guidance principles** to steer the group's activities.
>
> ➤ **Appoint a strong chair** who can help lead the group.
>
> ➤ **Provide training and support** for members where necessary.
>
> ➤ **Create working groups for projects** that report back to the wider group.
>
> ➤ **Adopt a champion** to help promote genuine service user involvement and raise the profile of the group.
>
> ➤ **Give the group time to evolve** it may need to find its feet and 'gel' before it becomes an effective body.
>
> ➤ **Build up links with external bodies** for example national organisations and networks.
>
> ➤ **Get the balance of membership right** try to foster ownership of the group.
>
> ➤ **Be clear about the group's role** to avoid confusion about membership and purpose.

Figure 4.1 Key ideas for establishing an effective user group.

> ➤ **Check participant's needs:** Ask all participants if they have any access requirements, e.g. a hearing loop, lip speakers and sign language interpreters. Equipment may need to be tested. Some people may need to bring a carer or a personal assistant with them.
>
> ➤ **Provide information:** Send an agenda in advance of the meeting which includes a short summary of the reason for the meeting and the items that will be discussed. Hold the meet at a convenient time and schedule in enough breaks.
>
> ➤ **Transport:** Provide advice about public transport and if necessary book travel arrangements. Explain where there is car parking. Send parking permits in advance.
>
> ➤ **Entrances:** Use buildings with good access, e.g. wide doorways and ground floor meeting rooms. Greet people at the entrance if possible. Put up clear signs to the meeting room.
>
> ➤ **Meeting rooms:** Natural lighting and well ventilated rooms at a comfortable temperature are preferable. Air-conditioning systems can be noisy.
>
> ➤ **Refreshments:** Provide drinking water. Clearly label food.

Figure 4.2 Key ideas for making events accessible.

highlights some main types of access issues that have been identified. Consideration should be paid to what the access issues for service users may be – this usually means contacting every individual in advance of a meeting or event and asking them what potential access issues are for them. In order to feel prepared service users are likely to need to know what the meeting is for and the type of topics that might be discussed.

> ➤ **Welcome:** Give a warm welcome to everyone, including any latecomers as they may have had a difficult trip.
> ➤ **House-keeping:** Explain where the toilets and fire exits are.
> ➤ **Introduction:** Briefly explain the purpose of the meeting and what the main agenda items are. Allow enough time for everyone to say something about themselves – for example who they are, what brings them to the meeting, what experience they have or what is important to them.
> ➤ **Ground rules:** Suggest ground rules and check whether everyone is happy with them.
> ➤ **Networking:** Allow time for people to ask each other questions and make connections.
> ➤ **The research:** Explain what the research is about and what the goals are allow time for questions and discussion.
> ➤ **Ways of working:** Decide how the meeting will be recorded and how everyone will keep informed and contribute ideas between meetings.
> ➤ **Sum-up:** Summarize the main things that have been discussed and decided. Agree next steps and who will be responsible for them.

Figure 4.3   Key ideas for a first meeting.

Written information about transport and maps should be provided to help people with the practical issues of getting to meetings and entering buildings.

Even if information has been provided in advance it is important to recognise that service users may not be familiar with research and they might be nervous about what the researchers expect of them, whether they will understand, or have anything to contribute. It is essential to put service users at ease by giving them a warm and friendly welcome when they first arrive. Making service users feel physically secure and comfortable will help to make service user involvement a success. Some ideas are summarised in Figure 4.3.

Don't forget how important it is for people to know who else is present at any meeting. Make sure there is plenty of time for individuals to introduce themselves to each other and find connections between one another. Make sure that right from the beginning service users feel they are involved. This will also help to avoid a 'them and us' situation where researchers are doing all the talking. Consider using a simple 'getting to know you exercise' such as asking individuals to introduce the person sitting next to them to other members of the group.

Research environments may not always be the best working environment for service user involvement. Service users may feel it is easier or feel more comfortable to access public buildings, such as a local community centre or library that has meeting rooms. Meetings can also be held in hotels or commercial venues if this has been budgeted for. It is advisable to start meetings after rush hour and when travel passes can be used.

Nursing and healthcare research often involves working with service users who have recent experience of clinical environments, such as in the following case study (Box 4.1).

Box 4.1   Managing diverse expectations

Case study

Jenny Laws, Researcher Durham University

My name is Jenny. I am a researcher and teaching fellow in the Faculty of Social Sciences and Health at Durham University. I have an interest in public involvement in research. In my master's and doctoral research I have been working with mental health service users on issues about recovery, employment and training. I also have personal experience of using mental health services.

Issue/Scenario: 'Whose side are you on?'

In 2006 we set up a service user self help group for people who had recently experienced in-patient psychiatric care, many of whom had found difficulties in engaging with conventional services or who did not automatically accept medical explanations for their distress. The aim was to use participatory approaches to provide a platform where service users could access peer-support and advocacy in a less clinical environment than the hospital.

Members enjoyed taking part in the project but found certain elements of academic practice frustrating and unexpected. One issue was that participants objected to risk assessment measures required by the university and disliked being described as a 'vulnerable population' – a term which they felt did not match the 'empowering' philosophy of the group. A particular condition of ethical agreement for the research was that I should not undertake research on anyone who was currently detained under the mental health act (a legal requirement, given concerns about such individuals' capacities to give 'informed consent'). Group members felt that this restriction jeopardised the autonomy of the support group and felt such individuals should not be excluded if they wanted to be involved. Both members of the group and members of the relevant ethics committee had difficulty in understanding the other's perspective.

Doing participatory research implies being 'on side' with research participants' agendas and priorities; yet integrating this with the wider political and intellectual environment of the university is not always easy. The above scenario ended with a compromise – I would discuss and collect general ideas *with* the service user group as a whole (so that everyone had a say) but, to meet the University's needs, I would not undertake any research *on* individual in-patients. Both sides were okay with this and this was actually a better fit with wanting to use a partnership approach in the research.

Key issues to be aware of:

- Service users are often very keen to get involved because they want to see direct improvements in services and have powerful personal insights to share. Expectations and enthusiasm of both service users and research organisations can be high at the start – it can be very exciting … but then challenges come along.
- Service users' views about what should happen in the research can 'collide' with the types of language, theory bases, ethical frameworks, bureaucracy and guidelines that are used in research environments.
- Language can be particularly sensitive when working with members of politicised service user movements. Terms like 'vulnerable groups' can undermine participatory values if this is not how participants define themselves.
- There can be situations where the researcher needs to face these challenges, break down the issue and look at what can be done to resolve it. For example, changing the wording of a document, being clearer about who can be involved and why, explaining what type of data can and can't be collected and by whom.

Helpful ideas:

- Keep a dialogue open. Just because there are different expectations and challenges it doesn't mean a compromise can't be found.
- It is important to keep a positive relationship between yourself, the research organisation and the service users involved. Be diplomatic and explain what the challenges are to everyone involved if it seems tensions are arising.
- Be clear to separate ethics and beliefs (what you as a researcher believe personally is right or good) from wider legal/time/financial restraints imposed by the research context. Sometimes it is okay to say, 'I'd love to, but I can't.'
- Try to work towards a range of outputs that take into consideration what is important to service users and academic requirements.

> Make an effort to arrive on time

> Switch off your mobile phone

> Be ready to introduce yourself

> Try to speak up so that everyone can hear

> Use plain and simple language

> Respect that each person has something to offer to the meeting

> Give others a chance to speak

> If you have a question or something to say indicate to the chair

> If you don't understand ask

> Agree what will be recorded and what is to be kept private

Figure 4.4   Ground rules for meetings.

Sometimes these experiences have been negative and service users may feel uncomfortable returning to a clinical setting. It may be more acceptable to find an alternative location to meet, if it is practical and safe to do so. It can also be important for service users who are receiving treatment to keep their role as a patient separate from their role as a service user involved in research. Researchers should consult service users about the type of locations and working environments that are acceptable to them.

Developing ground rules with service users helps to establish a preferred way of working and respect between group members. Figure 4.4 provides some key points for ground rules that can be discussed and adapted by research teams to suit their own preferences and needs.

Establishing a way of working also means finding out how everyone would like to be kept informed and contribute ideas outside of meetings. Find out whether service users want to exchange contact details and decide who will communicate information about the work between group members, or to those who cannot attend. In a buddy system service users have an allocated partner with whom they share any information or thoughts about the research.

Roles and responsibilities

Service users can take on different roles in the research, for example, as a:

- *Service user researcher*: A service user who designs and leads research studies.
- *Co-researcher/member of the research team*: Individual service users are appointed to contribute to designing, undertaking or evaluating the research.
- *Service user advisor*: Individual service users provide advice on specific aspects of the research as and when needed.

Box 4.2   Example role description for a member of a service user reference group

Service user with experience of cancer care

Purpose of role:

- To be an active member of the Service User Reference Group and contribute skills and knowledge about cancer care to the research study

This group member will:

- Be familiar with cancer services provided locally
- Have an understanding of the perspectives of patients receiving radiotherapy
- Have personal experience of being referred for radiotherapy treatment or receiving radiotherapy treatment in the last five years

Main responsibilities:

- To contribute to the design of an interview schedule about experiences of radiotherapy.
- To work with other members of the research team to analyse interview data from participants who are currently receiving/or have recently received radiotherapy.
- To work with other members of the research team to produce dissemination materials which meet the information needs of people who are offered radiotherapy treatment.

Each group member will:

- Attend meetings of the Service User Reference group (6–8 over a year).
- Read information that is sent before a meeting
- Read and consider summaries of meetings/action points
- Follow requirements for ethical working as explained by the researchers
- Be available for one-to-one discussion with members of the research team if necessary
- Participate in feedback and reflection about being involved in the research
- Declare any conflicts of interest or issues of concern that might arise in the research

---

Box 4.3   Example of service user responsibilities

General responsibilities:

- To be an active participant in the research by sharing thoughts and ideas with researchers and other service users involved
- To develop good working relationships with other service users and members of the research team
- To support others involved in the research, for example participate in a buddy system
- To read information that is sent before a meeting
- To read and consider summaries of meetings/action points
- To follow any requirements for ethical working as explained by the researchers, for example treating research data as confidential
- To participate in feedback and reflection about involvement

Specific responsibilities:

- To contribute to the design of the research or research tools
- To work on focused aspects of the research, for example undertaking research interviews
- To work on the analysis or interpretation of results
- To work on producing dissemination materials
- To contribute to writing-up case studies or lay summaries
- To review research reports or materials

- *Chair or member of a service user advisory group*: Service users are invited to be members of a group that works in collaboration with the research team.
- *Service user member of a research advisory group*: Individual service users are invited to join a group of other researchers and service users to provide advice to the research team.
- *Lay reviewer*: Service users are invited to critically review research outputs, for example reports or guidelines.

Some researchers and service users find it useful to develop a formal 'job description' to define what a service user's role is in the research (see for example, Box 4.2). In other situations it is more appropriate to allow the role to emerge over time as it becomes clearer what unique skills and knowledge an individual can contribute to the research.

The types of responsibilities that service users involved in the research will have should be made clear so that these can be discussed and agreed as early on as possible. Responsibilities might be general or specific, or a combination of both as illustrated by (Box 4.3).

Legal and ethical issues

Depending on the nature of the research and the type of service user involvement different legal and ethical issues will apply. In most situations it will be necessary for researchers

---

Box 4.4   Legislation relating to service user involvement in research

Duty of confidentiality

The common law duty of confidentiality requires that information is not disclosed without the consent of the individual, other than where required by legislation or where there is a robust public interest justification for disclosure. The person disclosing the information must be able to show that they have balanced the benefits of releasing the information with the rights of the individuals concerned and maintaining public trust in a confidential service.

The Data Protection Act 1998

Information about an individual must not be disclosed to other people, unless there is a legal or other overriding legitimate reason to share the information. The Data Protection Act makes it an offence for other people to obtain this personal data without authorisation.

Informed consent

Consent must be sought from a person before information about their care can be divulged to third parties. There are exceptions to this rule if the clinician thinks that, in the absence of consent, the person or other persons are put at risk. In such cases, they may waive this right and provide the information to third parties.

---

to discuss general principles of confidentiality, data protection and informed consent with service users who are participating in the research (Box 4.4).

Always consult a research ethics committee if you are in any doubt about what the ethical issues are. General issues are outlined in Chapter 3 ('Research ethics and governance' section). Specific types of ethical issues that can arise when working with different groups of service users are discussed in more detail in Chapters 5–8.

Training and support

It is considered good practice to offer service users training as part of being involved in research. Training can range in formality and duration to include:

- Participating in an interactive session, possibly with the researchers who the service users will be working with, to learn about the research and the types of methods and techniques that will be used.
- Attending a course that has been designed specifically to introduce service users to the principles of research.
- Formally undertaking a certified research methods course (not specifically designed for service users).
- Registering for personal study towards a degree or higher qualification with the backing of members of the research team.

Different types of training require different levels of commitment, time and financial support. Training must be appropriate for the level of service user involvement in the research and the roles and responsibilities that service users will take on. It is also important to remember that service users' experience and knowledge of research can vary considerably and that different people prefer to learn in different ways (Ormrod 1999).

In the UK guidelines for service user training have been developed from the research findings of the TRUE project (Training for Service User Involvement in Health and Social Care Research). The main guidelines (Lockey et al. 2004) are intended primarily for people who plan to provide training to service user researchers. However the extended guidelines also provide information for commissioners of training/research, researchers, service users involved in planning of training, and participants in training. The following box summarises these guidelines as action points for training of service users in research (Box 4.5).

Box 4.5   Training for service user involvement in health and social care research

Before training

- Trainers should be able to demonstrate competence, knowledge and understanding of service user involvement generally, and have sufficient knowledge of the service user group the training is aimed at
- Trainers should work with relevant service users and/or service user groups to plan the content, style and delivery of the training and the best environment to deliver the training
- Budget for extra costs that may be involved including transport, accommodation, and payment
- Identify what the most appropriate training methods are, for example role play, practice examples, factual information, learning on the job or a combination
- Plan to include informal learning opportunities, where people can share experiences, build confidence, learn from each other and have fun
- If appropriate, relate the training to a planned role/activity that will be accessible to participants following training
- Ensure that the language to be used is clear and free of jargon
- If using external trainers ensure they are able to provide suitable training
- Provide information to participants in advance about aims and objectives of the research, aims and objectives of the training and personal time investment that will be required
- Allow enough time in the timetable for a flexible and responsive training approach
- Ensure the venue is accessible and comfortable for all participants, provide a map and arrange transport if necessary, and provide refreshments and comfort breaks
- Ensure any payments for attendance or expenses are made promptly
- If appropriate provide a certificate of attendance or accreditation
- Plan to collect participants' feedback about the training

During training

- Make participants feel welcome
- Communicate clear aims and objectives
- Find out at the beginning how people view themselves and how they like to be referred to
- Make sure everyone's contribution is recognised and acknowledged
- Make use of learning methods that suit everyone
- Make it clear to participants that they should ask if clarification is needed

After training

- Collect feedback from participants
- Thank participants for their willingness to take part in the training and award certificates or acknowledge their achievements
- Allow time after the training to develop the research
- Provide some continuity for people, so that the contact does not end abruptly when the training ends
- Explore with participants their further training needs and wishes
- Reflect on your own role in providing training

Communication

For any research study or programme of work it can be beneficial to develop a concise written communication strategy (no more than a few pages of text) that can be shared with anyone involved in the research. Developing a written strategy can encourage those involved in the research to find ways to:

- Develop good working relationships
- Engage people in the research
- Promote the research, its aims and objectives
- Disseminate the findings and implement changes

Communication should be thought of as a two-way process that can follow a number of channels, such as:

- Between members of the research team (which may include service users)
- Between service users who are involved in the research
- To participants in the research
- To stakeholders in the research, for example commissioners, advisory group members
- To research communities, healthcare practitioners and managers
- To local communities and the general public

Communication is a key area where service users can help to make the research more accessible to different audiences. Working together researchers and service users can identify potential target audiences, decide what type of information to share with each audience, what you would like the audience to do as a result, when to communicate, and how best to communicate, as illustrated by Figure 4.5.

There are a range of direct or indirect communication methods, as depicted by Figure 4.6. Researchers may be used to providing written materials, such as research reports and academic papers to research audiences. Other methods are likely to be more effective for communicating with non-academic audiences, such as newsletters and short

> ➤ **Who you want to reach:** identify your audiences and who would benefit from this information.
> ➤ **What you want to share:** establish what you want to say and whether the message needs to be tailored for specific audiences. Focus on positive as well as negative themes for a balanced view.
> ➤ **Why you want to share the information:** be clear about what you want to achieve and what you want your audience to do as a result.
> ➤ **When and where you are going to communicate:** choose a time to reach your audience when they are likely to be most receptive. Break the activity down into 'bite-size' stages. Inform audiences about these as they take place, as well as after to help prepare them and establish a positive relationship.
> ➤ **How you will share your information:** consider the best formats to reach each audience. This will vary according to their needs and circumstances.

Figure 4.5   Developing a communication strategy.

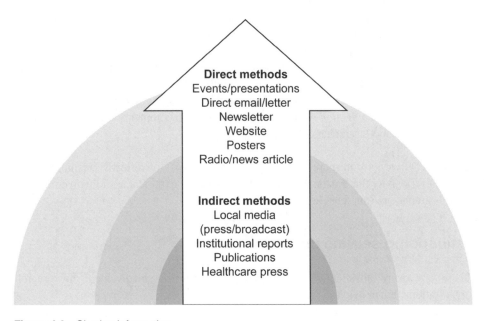

Direct methods
Events/presentations
Direct email/letter
Newsletter
Website
Posters
Radio/news article

Indirect methods
Local media
(press/broadcast)
Institutional reports
Publications
Healthcare press

Figure 4.6   Sharing information.

articles in organisational magazines. Electronic media, such as web-based information, podcasts and digital video discs, can be very effective in reaching widespread audiences and for presenting the research in an interesting way. At conferences or events service users may wish to co-present sessions or co-facilitate workshops about the research.

Feedback and reflection

Feedback from the research team to service users who are involved is important for keeping people informed about how things are progressing and whether any changes in the research or involvement may need to be made. Ways of feeding back to service users can include sending written 'project updates' between meetings, summaries and action points, or newsletters. Feedback from service users to researchers can also be used to make sure that involvement is working well. Feedback is normally a positive and supportive process, but asking for feedback can sometimes raise sensitive or personal issues. Researchers should explain the type of feedback that would be helpful for them, such as requesting comments about ways of working, the research itself, or ideas for improvement.

In an everyday sense, reflection means 'looking back' on experiences so as to learn from them. Service users and researchers can make use of a range of reflective techniques as the research progresses, for example:

- *Reflective diaries*: written journals or video diaries about the research and how it is progressing. Service users may choose to share all or some of their personal reflections with other members of the group.
- *Interviews about involvement*: service users or researchers can interview each other about the strengths and weaknesses of working relationships.
- *Group discussions*: open discussions about the research or involvement.
- *Reflection and feedback forms*: individual self-completion forms which are provided to the research team. These could ask about what individuals think is important, what they have learnt, or what they will take away from their experiences to share with others.
- *Suggestion boxes/reflection boards*: anonymous written comments are read out to other service users and researchers.

In Chapter 9 we look in more detail at the different types of reflective techniques and forms of reflexivity that can be used to examine personal experiences of involvement and organisational environments for involvement.

Embedding service user involvement

There are many advantages to developing service user involvement in research organisations. It can help to:

- Spread service user involvement beyond the project level which could achieve better research across whole programmes or research organisations.
- Grow research relationships between researchers and service users that build links between research studies, practice and service development.
- Develop connections between research institutions and service user organisations to support future research and development.
- Build expertise and knowledge about service user involvement across research units, departments and organisations.

- Develop best practices for ways of working and support systems for service users.
- Create a critical capacity of researchers who can provide peer-to-peer support for less experienced researchers about working with service users.

As illustrated by the following case study (Box 4.6), embedding involvement in learning organisations can involve different types of organisational and practical barriers. Making connections, developing good working relationships and providing support for service users can help to maximise the value of involvement. Of course there are also advantages to collaborating across organisations and geographical areas (Davies and Evans 2010).

Box 4.6   Embedding service user involvement in learning organisations

Case study

Prof. Colin Torrance, Dr. Keith Weeks and Christine Wilson

We are part of a research team at the University of Glamorgan investigating the use of clinical simulation and virtual learning environments to educate healthcare professionals including undergraduate nursing students. Building on previous research and development work undertaken by the Simulation Centre team (http://hesas.glam.ac.uk/simulation) we are advancing a model of pedagogical practice and clinical education that employs the simulated clinical environment (1–5).

Improving the authenticity of clinical simulation – A work in progress

Clinical simulation is a rapidly developing educational technology which can help students to master clinical skills and reasoning in a controlled and safe environment. Students can be offered high risk or low frequency clinical interactions that provide the opportunity to practice and rehearse skills in situations where it would be impractical, unsafe and/or unethical to do so with real patients (6). We believe that more authentic, and therefore more effective, clinical simulation experiences can be achieved if we involve patients and carers in the research, design and undertaking of clinical simulation. Part of our current research programme questions how we can better embed the voice and experience of patients and carers into the learning activities that take place in the clinical simulation centre (CSC). This is an important but currently unexplored area of research that offers the potential to yield benefits for both patients and health professionals alike.

The educational model takes a constructivist based learning approach, articulated within a cognitive apprenticeship framework (7). Assessment and evaluation activities are further informed by Gulikers' five dimensional framework of authentic assessment (8). This dynamic model underpins the Faculty's authentic health professional educational programmes. Maintaining a realistic environment is an essential component of this model. This not only means having a manikin device capable of adequately reproducing the patient condition, but also creating a learning environment that looks and feels like the real world.

Using a simulated learning environment where patients and carers have a strong voice, our aim is to more closely align healthcare professionals for fitness for award and fitness for practice activities by assisting learners to adapt to their role as individual practitioners and multi-disciplinary team members. Our approach is to apply grounded theory and exclusive participatory techniques to embed the service user and carer perspective into the various authentic elements of the simulated and virtual reality paradigms, including the physical context and environment, the authentic social context, the authentic learning activities and the feedback and assessment context.

Issues to be aware of:

- Embedding involvement in learning organisations can involve different types of organisational and practical barriers.
- In capturing and maintaining a realistic clinical environment we need to harness and combine professional and lay perspectives. Otherwise, all we will achieve is a healthcare environment best suited to the professional rather than the patient – it is the authentic patient perspective that is so often missing from this type of education and research.

Helpful ideas:

- Establish links with different voluntary and public sector organisations. For example, we have established links with the Dignified Revolution, various Cancer Trusts, Chronic illness organisations and the Welsh Centre for Equality and Diversity in Healthcare.
- Develop a data base of people willing to be involved in the education and research currently being undertaken in the organisation (or specifically in clinical simulation).
- Invite patients and carer groups to be involved in specific activities and monitor the impact on quality outcomes.
- Provide training for service user and carer groups in order to maximise the value of their input.
- Establish novel participatory events within the simulated learning environment such as a 'Living Library' (see Chapter 7 of this book).
- Capture learning to increase student learning using DVD and studio code and to strengthen feedback and reflective practice.
- Take a grounded theory approach.

(1) Weeks, K.W., Lyne. P., and Torrance, C. (2000) Written drug dosage errors made by students: the threat to clinical effectiveness and the need for a new approach. *Clinical Effectiveness in Nursing*, 4, 20–2.
(2) Weeks, K.W. (2001) Setting a foundation for the development of medication dosage calculation problem solving skills among novice nursing students. The role of constructivist learning approaches and a computer based. *UWCM Nursing, Health and Social Care Research Unit Discussion Paper* (ISBN: 1 903847 036). Cardiff: UWCM.
(3) Weeks, K.W., Lyne, P., Moseley, L., and Torrance, C. (2001) The strive for clinical effectiveness in medication dosage calculation problem solving skills: the role of constructivist learning theory in the design of a computer based 'Authentic World' learning environment. *Clinical Effectiveness in Nursing*, 5, 18–25.
(4) Weeks, K.W. and Lowes, L. (2006) Researching your own clients/students. In: Lyne, P. and Allan, D. (eds) *The Reality of Nursing Research*. Oxford: Routledge Falmer.
(5) Weeks, K.W. (2007) No more 'chalk and talk': teaching drug calculation skills for the real world. *Safer Healthcare*, Retrieved 26 August, 2007, from http://www.authenticworld.co.uk/downloads/press/saferhealthcare.pdf' Authentic World' learning environment. Unpublished PhD, University of Glamorgan, Pontypridd.
(6) Torrance, C., Wilson, C., and Mansell, I. (2009) The ethical implications of using patients to educate student nurses, Unpublished, University of Glamorgan, Pontypridd.
(7) Collins, A., Brown, R., and Newman, S. (1989) Cognitive apprenticeship: teaching the crafts of reading, writing, and mathematics. In: Resnick, L. (ed) *Learning and Instruction. Essays in Honor of Robert Glaser*. Hillsdale, NJ: Lawrence Erlbaum Associates.
(8) Gulikers, J.T.M., Bastiaens, T.J., and Kirscner, P.A. (2004) A five-dimensional framework for authentic assessment. *Educational Technology Research and Development*, 52 (3): 67–86.

Key principles for practice

- Make connections with service users through existing research relationships, clinical relationships, local services, public advertisements or approaches to service user organisations and community groups. Provide clear information about who is being approached, the purpose of the research and opportunities for involvement.
- Consult service users about the type of locations and working environments that are acceptable to them. Provide people with equal opportunity to participate fully in the research by helping them feel they are able to understand, communicate, and participate in a way that suits them.
- Discuss and agree the types of roles and responsibilities that service users involved in the research will have as early on as possible.
- Discuss general principles of confidentiality, data protection and informed consent with service users who are participating in the research.
- Offer service users appropriate training as part of being involved in the research.
- Think about how you communicate in relation to developing working relationships, engaging people in the research, promoting the research aims and objectives, and disseminating findings.
- Provide feedback to service users to keep people informed about how things are progressing. Ask for feedback from service users to make sure that involvement is working well, for example using reflective diaries, interviews, group discussions, feedback forms, suggestion boxes or reflection boards.
- Contribute to embedding service user involvement by spreading learning across programmes or research organisations, building expertise and developing best practice for ways of working and support systems.

References

Davies, R. and Evans, D. (2010) *Public involvement in research: How Can Organisations Collaborate to Improve Involvement?* University of the West of England, Bristol on Behalf of Fourteen Stakeholder Organisations in Bristol and the South West.

Lockey, R., Sitzia, J., Gillingham, T., Millyard, J., Miller, C., Ahmed, S., Beales, A., Bennett, C., Parfoot, S., Sigrist, G., and Sigrist, J. (2004) *Training for Service User Involvement in Health and Social Care Research: A Study of Training Provision and Participants' Experiences (The TRUE Project).* Worthing: Worthing and Southlands Hospitals NHS Trust.

Ormrod, J. (1999) *Human Learning*, 3rd edn. Upper Saddle River, NJ: Prentice-Hall.

Rhodes, P., Nocon, A., Wright, J., and Harrison, S. (2001) Involving patients in research. Setting up a service users' advisory group. *Journal of Management in Medicine*, 15 (2): 167–71.

Rhodes, P., Nocon, A., Booth, M., Chowdrey, M., Fabian, A., Neville, L., Fagir, M., and Walgrove, T. (2002) A service users' research advisory group from the perspective of both service users and researchers. *Health & Social Care in the Community*, 10 (5): 402–409.

Part II

Learning

Chapter 5

Patients, clients and carers

Key summary points

- *Patients who are receiving health care*: There are many reasons and ways to bring a patient's viewpoint to all kinds of healthcare issues. Involving patients who are receiving health care in research requires striking a fine balance between the ethical duties of providing care and support, and achieving involvement that is worthwhile and meaningful.
- *People who are very sick*: Although people who are very sick are sometimes described as 'vulnerable', if researchers put in place practical and ethical protections it is unethical to exclude such individuals from research if they wish to participate.
- *People with rare clinical conditions*: When seeking to involve people with rare clinical conditions in research, patients generally express great enthusiasm about improving care or services but researchers need to explain the scale and pace of improvements that can be made.
- *People who find it difficult to access services*: Barriers to service use and involvement in research can include: disability, age, ethnicity, sexuality, people with severe learning disabilities and/or communication impairments, mental health problems, homelessness, substance abuse, geographical isolation, and refugee/asylum seeker status.
- *People who do not have the capacity to consent*: In the case of some seldom-heard groups, their right to give informed consent has typically been ignored, and unwarranted assumptions have been made about their lack of legal competence. Research evidence and changing conceptions of individual rights have led to statutory changes which recognise the capacity to give informed consent is a continuum, and a person's capacity to make decisions may vary depending on the specific topic or area of life under consideration.
- *Carers*: Like service users, carers are a diverse group. Their views tend to differ from the interests of clinical research professionals, as well as the views of those they care for. Challenges of involving carers in research can include recognising the benefits and different perspectives that carers bring to research, practical issues of identifying carers to be involved, and finding time away from caring.

Handbook of Service User Involvement in Nursing and Healthcare Research, First Edition.
Elizabeth Morrow, Annette Boaz, Sally Brearley and Fiona Ross.
© 2012 Elizabeth Morrow, Annette Boaz, Sally Brearley and Fiona Ross.
Published 2012 by Blackwell Publishing Ltd.

Patients who are receiving health care

There are many reasons and ways to bring a patient's viewpoint to all kinds of healthcare issues. Often patients who are receiving treatment or care feel it is important that they are asked about their experiences and that professionals take their views on board. Similarly, patients who choose to participate in research may see it as a way of improving treatment or services for others and therefore have an expectation that their contributions will be acted upon. For researchers, involving patients in research could mean gaining a better understanding of the issues at hand and what is important to patients.

Involving patients who are receiving health care in research requires striking a fine balance between the ethical duties of providing care and support, and achieving involvement that is accessible and meaningful. As illustrated by the case study (Box 5.1), the decision to participate in research can feel like an added burden to patients at a time when they are vulnerable, but it can also be a great opportunity if it is approached in the right way. Patients receiving treatment or care may be under greater physical and emotional stress than normal, which could mean that the research methods that are used need to be adapted to include additional time for patients to rest or to defer their participation on a particular day. Patients receiving treatment or care may feel that their care will be affected if they do not participate in the research, even if this is not the case (Newman and Kaloupek 2004). The issues can be even more sensitive or complex if the same healthcare professional providing care to a patient is also undertaking the research.

There are other groups of people who may not necessarily be considered as 'patients receiving care' even though they come into regular contact with health services. For example, women who are pregnant, in labour or breast feeding also require special consideration (National Childbirth Trust 2001). In the same respect, people who are eligible for screening or immunisation, or have attended such programmes, may not perceive themselves as being patients. People who have received treatment for cancer in the past and who are still registered for check-ups may prefer to be called 'survivors' or 'patient advocates' if they become involved in research.

In recent years patient surveys have become a popular way of collecting information from people that have come into contact with health services. The extent and volume of data now routinely being collected are significant in the light of moves towards increased service user involvement in research. Surveys could be about patient satisfaction, broader aspects of the patient experience, along with perceptions of safety and effectiveness for example (Bate and Robert 2003). In the UK, national guidance sets out best practice in terms of collecting, analysing and using patient feedback (Department of Health 2008). A potential shortcoming of patient surveys is that they represent a low level of involvement – professionals design the survey and set the questions to be asked. Thus, when planning patient surveys careful thought needs to be given to asking the right questions at the right level, for example ward level, division, department, clinic, and clinician (The Healthcare Commission 2006). It is essential to be clear about what the aim of data collection is, for example a patient survey to inform service re-design would need to ask about patient expectations and suggestions for improvements to existing services. In other situations it would be more useful to have consistency of questions over time for comparability, benchmarking and showing progress.

Box 5.1   Service user involvement in clinical trials for breast cancer treatment

Case study

Hazel Thornton

I describe myself as an independent advocate for quality in research and health care. Prior to my involvement as a non-health professional in the research process, my husband and I ran a small irrigation company in the U.K.

'My route to involvement'

My 'Damascus Road' moment occurred in 1991 when circumstances forced me to recognise the uncertainty inherent in treatments offered; to realise that adequate, clear information ought to be available for public and patients; to appreciate that good quality research is essential, not optional; and recognise that everyone has a responsibility to support or contribute to that endeavour. My eye-opener was being invited to participate in the UK randomised trial for the management of screen-detected ductal carcinoma in situ (DCIS) of the breast. It led me to closely scrutinise the practical and ethical aspects of this proposition, and the benefit/harm ratio of population screening. My own research led me eventually to:

- Campaign for better research generally;
- Advocate for active patient and public involvement in the whole research process;
- Ensure that better information be made available for patients and citizens; and
- For better public education about research (1).

I realised that my experience was of social significance. Numerous other eligible women who had had abnormalities discovered at breast screening would be in the same predicament of being required to make a decision whether to consent or not to participate in this contentious and inadequate trial. This led me to write to my surgeon, to write to all the members of the trial management committee, to seek publication of my concerns (2), and to begin to inform myself more fully about DCIS, research processes and other relevant matters. As a result, various dialogues were initiated with health professionals who were helpful because they saw benefit in pursuing these topics with a lay person, and in the mutually educative and practical potential of more generally engaging in such exchanges.

This activity, together with exposure in the journals and other resultant exchanges, led to various invitations. In December 1991, Professor Michael Baum wrote to say that he would like to establish a dialogue and to meet. In 1993, Sir Iain Chalmers invited me to give a seminar at Green College Oxford for the Clinical Trials Service Unit and the UK Cochrane Centre. I chose as my subject: *Is there a moral obligation for patients to join randomised controlled trials?* Subsequently, I took this seminar to hospital venues in London, Edinburgh, Manchester, Bristol, Mount Vernon, and to King's College, London. *The Lancet* invited me to speak to an international audience of breast cancer specialists at their first conference in Bruges, *The Challenge of Breast Cancer,* in April 1994, on the topic *The patient's role in research* (3). Dr Imogen Evans chaired this plenary session, with Professor Michael Baum as overall chair of the morning.

Professor Baum then suggested that we should jointly found a combined health professional/patient working group. We set up the *Consumers' Advisory Group for Clinical Trials (CAG-CT)* (Registered Charity No. 1051813) in September 1994 in order 'to initiate, promote, facilitate and produce quality research that met the needs and interests of patients, the public and health professionals by advancing education in medical research methodology'. This activity was given endorsement by the House of Commons in 1995 (4). Research organisations described the CAG-CT as a 'facilitator for progress'.

Key issues:

- Research is everyone's business!
- There is no single correct way.
- Participate in 'equal' dialogues to iterate and collaborate.
- Service users have individual skills to bring as one of a team, not as a special category.

Helpful ideas:

- I have found many ways to discuss and demonstrate the potential value of bringing a patient's viewpoint to all kinds of medical and research endeavours (5). My own involvement led to invitations to write for journals, to be a member of trial management teams, to comment on research applications, to comment on patient information, to review papers for journals, to give conference presentations, to assist in training courses, to comment for the media, and to join editorial boards.
- This was my route to involvement. There are many different and valuable ways to suit all types of people: within organised structures; individually; or as participants in facilitated qualitative research.

(1) Evans, I., Thornton, H., and Chalmers, I. (2006) *Testing Treatments – Better Research for Better Healthcare*. The British Library. ISBN 0-7123-4909-X. Now re-issued by Pinter and Martin 2010. Also available without charge from the James Lind Library website www.jameslindlibrary.org in English and various translations.
(2) Thornton, H.M. (1992) Breast cancer trials: a patient's viewpoint. *Lancet*, 339: 44–45.
(3) Thornton, H. (July 1995) The patient's role in research (Paper given at *The Lancet "Challenge of Breast Cancer"Conference*, Brugge, April 1994.) In *Health Committee Third Report. Breast Cancer Services. Volume II. Minutes of Evidence and Appendices*. London: HMSO, pp. 112–4.
(4) House of Commons Health Committee. (July 1995) *Third Report Breast Cancer Services, Volume II, Minutes of Evidence and Appendices*. London: HMSO.
(5) Thornton, H. (2006) Patients and health professionals working together to improve clinical research: where are we going? *European Journal of Cancer*, 42: 2454–8, plus Appendix A. online at doi:10.1016/j.ejca.2006.05.022

A range of methods and techniques have been devised to attain 'near real time' feedback from patients. These include comment cards, self-completion/paper-based surveys and personal digital assistants (PDAs); delivered either by researchers, clinical staff, audit teams and/or hospital volunteers. Different information technologies have been developed such as handheld patient experience trackers, which are used within clinical settings to reach large numbers of patients. Using such tools can be very effective for gaining information but they could be perceived as being a very low level of patient involvement – consultation rather than active involvement (as discussed in 'Representation' section). Furthermore, when patient experience data are collected at the point of care delivery there are practical issues of the burden on staff of collecting such information, as well as ethical issues of bias, neutrality and providing support for patient's clinical needs rather than research and service improvement tasks. Reviewing complaints and other sources of patient feedback – for example involving patient support groups – can help to explore wider patient attitudes and the extent to which patient's expectations about a service are met. Collecting in-depth patient experience data needs to be balanced with having both appropriate methods and resources to do so, to be able to evaluate changes that have been made and, ultimately, to show evidence of service improvement (Bate and Robert 2007). As well as theoretical and practical limitations of relying on patient surveys of satisfaction for informing service improvement work (Williams 1994), variations in people's expectations of what kind of service they should receive can be considerable, and factors like geographical location, age, gender and ethnicity can all impact on the kinds of responses received (Wise 2009).

A common issue in relation to patient experience data is whose views are, and are not, being represented. Hence, it is important to consider different response levels and the clinical significance of different patients' experiences, for example the experiences of patients who undergo rare high-risk procedures may be more clinically important than those who undergo routine low-risk procedures (Cleary 1999). There are also issues about the comparability of patient experience data and analysis across different population bases, such as between different cultural groups and geographical areas.

People who are very sick

People who are very sick are sometimes referred to as 'vulnerable groups'. However, the problem with using this term is that it carries a lot of moral weight, and labelling people as vulnerable can actually close off conversation about their involvement in research (Beresford and Campbell 1994). Figure 5.1 illustrates some of the complexities of involving acutely ill patients in research. Despite these complexities researchers can take steps to involve patients who wish to participate – most importantly, being sensitive to the nature of the illness.

There may also be further issues for researchers to consider if people are receiving palliative care or are near end-of-life. Such individuals are likely to experience changing priorities and views depending on their personal circumstances (Addington-Hall 2002). However, some researchers have argued that research in near end-of-life care is constrained more by pragmatic, social, cultural and financial constraints than ethical issues (Small and Rhodes 2000; Cotterell et al. 2005). They suggest that when normally accepted and ethically sound protections are in place, exclusion of patients with far advanced disease or serious injury who want to participate in research is itself unethical (Agrawal 2003; Fine 2003; Abma 2005). The following case study (Box 5.2)

Complexities of acute illness	Involvement challenges
Intensity and complexity of the illness	Sensitivity to the nature of the illness
Co-morbidity	Understanding of co-morbidities
Pain	Allowance for limited mobility
Fatigue	Assessment of level of concentration
Delirium or unconsciousness	Knowing when to withdraw/return
Frequent service/ward transfer	Keeping track of where patients are
Time for multiple Treatments/appointments	Flexible meetings (places/times)
Carer support	Working with carers to enable involvement
Family relationships	Respecting wishes of the family
Personal financial and social circumstances	Sensitivity to personal worries or concerns

Figure 5.1   Involving people with acute illness.

Box 5.2   Hearing the voices of those who are very sick

Case study

Sally Crowe

I am a consultant in Patient and Public Involvement (PPI). Before that I was a nurse and public health practitioner. For the last 15 years I have enjoyed working with patient and carer groups and multi-professional partnerships exploring all aspects of involvement. My current interests are in the impact of PPI and working with involved patients and the public on a one-to-one (coaching) basis.

Devising and designing a searchable database of patient experiences

In 2004 the GUS (Great Universal Stores) Charitable Trust funded a project called Partnership for Research in ME/CFS (Myalgic Encephalophathy/Chronic Fatigue Syndrome) or PRIME for short. It was a collaboration of patients, clinicians and researchers working to improve understanding of patients' experiences with this complex disease. A key output of the project was a patient experience resource for researchers to access to inform their work, particularly the narratives of people severely affected by the condition.

A steering group of people invited from research, clinical, web design and patient organisations met regularly to plan the project and oversee progress. The first meeting highlighted the tensions and challenges of working in an area where patients had felt marginalised by the NHS, and were cautious of new endeavours. Good working relationships were developed via meetings, email and telephone contact and regular consultations about aspects of the project. At meetings, special arrangements were made for people with visual and cognitive impairment. Expenses were always paid in cash and on the day.

The principal challenge for this project was to create a searchable database of primary data around patients' experiences. Interviews with 40 people with CFS/ME generated rich data for the project. Interviewing had to be sensitive to the needs of people with visual, auditory and cognitive impairments. The involvement of patient groups enabled us to be prepared for such eventualities.

The database needed to be sensitive to different types of searching behaviour, that is users might want to look at young people's experiences, or be interested in particular symptoms and aspects of the condition; others would want the whole story. Developing the database website was a collaborative effort, with the involvement of service users adding value at different stages of development.

Key issues to be aware of:

• Service users can be advocates for the project at all stages – for example helping to recruit interviewees and prepare interview guides, helping to plan and host research workshops to generate content for the website, and visiting service user groups and events to publicise the resource.
• Service users can provide feedback on pilot versions of a database or a website – which helps to improve accessibility and usability.
• In this study service users were involved in a rigorous process for anonymising and checking the 'patient stories' without distorting the original experiences.

Helpful ideas:

• Be clear about what you want service users to contribute to your research. This will make your initial approach more cohesive and attractive. Our vision was incomplete when we started the project and it was difficult for everyone to share it.
• Keep in mind the practical and emotional aspects of involvement. We were aware of some people finding involvement exhausting because of their condition; we got better at pacing our activities.

> - Invest time and effort in building a service user group. Spend time establishing team relationships and finding strengths. Confront the challenges and use the whole group to find solutions.
> - The politics in ME/CFS are interesting in themselves; the service users were the best at helping us understand the issues and deal with them.

presents some helpful ideas for overcoming ethical and practical challenges of involving people who are very sick in research.

People with rare clinical conditions

A key issue to be aware of when seeking to involve people with rare clinical conditions in research is that patients generally express great enthusiasm about improving care or services but there is a danger of raising expectations about the scale and pace of improvements that can be made. A patient's suggestions for improvements will not necessarily be supported by healthcare professionals or taken up by health services. Of course, this point applies to all research but it can be particularly the case where people have rare illnesses where little research is being undertaken. Researchers need to be clear and open about the limitations which surround the research and what might realistically be achieved. As illustrated by the following case study (Box 5.3), research can be about helping people to live their lives, as well as seeking cures to their illnesses.

People who find it difficult to access services

Some people find it difficult to access mainstream health services for various reasons. These people are less likely to be heard by service professionals and decision-makers. Barriers to service use and involvement in research can include:

- Disability
- Age
- Ethnicity
- Sexuality
- People with severe learning disabilities and/or communication impairments
- Mental health problems
- Homelessness
- Substance abuse
- Geographical isolation
- Refugee or asylum seeker status

These groups of people are sometimes also referred to as 'hard to reach' groups, though this term has been criticised for implying that there is something about these people that

Box 5.3   Involving people with chronic and severe skin conditions in research

Case study

Dr Patricia Grocott, Reader Palliative Wound Care, King's College London

About 20 years ago now I was working in a clinical nursing role with patients suffering from chronic skin conditions. The patients I saw on a daily basis had different types of wounds. Some had lived with their conditions all of their lives, others were living with post-operative wounds or cancer-related wounds. I felt the care we could give was desperately inadequate because we just didn't have the right tools to be able to care for people with severe skin conditions. The wound dressings were too small or inflexible, and often did more harm than good to the patient's fragile skin causing pain and suffering. I moved into academic research because I felt it was the right place for me to strategically address some of the terrible problems with medical devices for wound care that I had observed in practice. I now work very closely with Elizabeth Pillay and other specialist clinicians at St Thomas' Hospital, members of industry, and members of DebRA (www.debra.org.uk) the national charity for people with the genetic skin blistering condition, epidermolysis bullosa (EB). Together we are working in partnership to understand the issues better and to develop new solutions to wound care.

Elizabeth Pillay, EB Nurse Consultant, Debra UK, St Thomas' Hospital London

I have worked with people with the skin fragility/blistering disorder EB for the last 16 years. People with the severe forms of the condition will live with extensive, life-long wounding. With no curative treatment possible, our role in the EB service is to offer the best available symptom management. Although the science of wound care has developed apace there is an absolute dearth of wound care products which are designed to meet the needs of those people with extensive, never-to-heal wounding. Our work with Patricia Grocott has brought the opportunity to think creatively and with academic rigour with the object of developing wound care solutions for the group who have palliative wound care needs. Excitingly, this partnership has included those at the 'sharp end', that is the patients and carers.

Helping people live as normally as possible

Chronic and extensive wounds can have an appalling impact on a person's ability to live a normal daily life. Their skin may never heal. It can be permanently painful to touch, fragile, leak exudates, and be prone to infection and odour. Getting the right sorts of dressings and care can make the difference between someone being confined to their bed or being able to do the things they want to.

Patricia: I remember distinctly one young woman who was dying from advanced breast cancer. She decided to try a yoga class to get some mental and spiritual release from her condition. The only dressings available were too small (20 × 20 cm) to cover the extensive broken skin across her chest and we had to overlap several single dressings. They began to fall away and the leaking wounds on her chest were exposed to the class. She was very distressed and did not return to the class even though the group was supportive and understanding.

Elizabeth: This kind of sad experience is all too often part of the day-to-day life of those people living with EB. They are frequently constrained in their choice of activity, not only as a result of the disabilities which result from having severe EB, but also by inadequate wound care products which may allow embarrassing leakage, slippage causing pain, and take many gruelling hours each day to apply fresh dressings. The cost to supply such inadequate products is often colossal both in terms of quality of life and financially. I am for instance working with a young man who was a postdoctoral researcher, who has had to sacrifice his career following a deterioration in the condition of his skin. As a consequence, he has to spend 4 painful hours each day with nurses and carers removing and applying a 'patchwork' of dressings. The pain caused by this procedure is such that large doses of opiates are required to achieve some level of pain control, and this combined with the time taken to change the dressings makes pursuing his promising career impossible for the foreseeable future.

As we see it, the role of the nurse is to help people live as normal a life as possible without pain or emotional distress – safe and secure dressings should be a standard that we can promise all patients.

Key issues to be aware of:

- Patients generally express great enthusiasm about improving medical devices and care when researchers ask them about their experiences. However, there is a danger of raising expectations about the scale and pace of improvements that can be made. New products or improvements will not necessarily be supported by the wound care industry or taken up by the health service.
- Product design and development in collaboration with patients needs to be undertaken with the utmost regard for their safety and well-being. Ethical responsibility, clinical duty of care, and informed consent are key issues to be aware of at every stage.

Helpful ideas:

- Working with patients who suffer chronic and severe conditions requires continuous open dialogue about their views, experiences and expectations for the work. Researchers must work closely with clinicians, patients and carers to make sure they are working to solve the right problems in the right way.
- Groundwork with service users to understand the issues, as well as piloting and testing of ideas, can be a slow iterative process but is more effective than designing an intervention without fully understanding the problem from the perspective of patients and clinicians who experience it on a daily basis.

makes their engagement with services difficult (Beresford and Campbell 1994). In fact, it can be that the barriers to involvement are more to do with social or geographical factors rather than to do with the individuals themselves, such as living in a rural location (Morgan et al. 2005). The term 'seldom-heard' places more of the emphasis on agencies to engage these service users, carers and potential service users. Chapter 7 looks in more depth at the barriers and the issues of involving seldom-heard groups in research.

People who do not have the capacity to consent

For some groups of people there may be ethical concern about the extent to which they are able to give informed consent to participate in research, or to be involved as partners in the research. Gaining informed consent is often a complex aspect of nursing and healthcare research processes because of the difficulty of establishing what a person should be 'informed' about in relation to any particular research study and their level of participation or involvement in it (RCN 2005). The term 'capacity to consent' is a legal term which relates to an individual's ability to make decisions (Chadwick 2001). While written consent is the usual method of recording informed consent in research, some people may be unable to read and/or write, and other methods of obtaining and recording informed consent may be more appropriate.

People who do not have the capacity to consent have the same rights as other members of society, including the right to choose whether to participate in research and the right to be protected from any undue risks from participation in research. Historically, people who do not have the capacity to consent have experienced disadvantage, overprotection and abuse. People with intellectual disabilities or dementia are such individuals who may be at risk of information not being provided at an appropriate level, or of not being able to understand or reason adequately about their participation. Their right to give informed consent has typically been ignored, and unwarranted assumptions have been made about their lack of legal competence. Research evidence and changing conceptions of individual rights have led to statutory changes which recognise the capacity to give informed consent is a continuum, and a person's capacity to make decisions may vary depending on the specific topic or area of life under consideration.

When seeking to involve people who do not have the capacity to consent in research researchers should ensure that:

- The research is well designed and focuses on an issue of significant importance to the people being involved;
- The capacity of an individual to give informed consent should be assessed on a case-by-case basis;
- The rights of people to make their own choices is respected, even if they are not able to give informed consent themselves;
- People are protected from undue risks, exploitation and abuse.

Researchers may also find it useful to include within the research team one or more individuals who are knowledgeable about and experienced in working with people who do not have the capacity to consent.

People who do not have the capacity to consent are not usually concerned about the implications of research for service development or public policy, but are more likely to be interested in what changes the research can bring about for them personally. It may be that people who do not have the capacity to consent have a tendency to comply with the perceived demands of an authority figure. However, even people with severe learning disabilities may be able to make decisions if given the opportunity and support to do so. For example, researchers may need to:

- Spend time explaining the meaning of abstract words and ideas;
- Provide information that is personalised to the individual's level of understanding;
- Revisit individuals several times to discuss ideas, because of shorter attention spans and reduced short-term memory;
- Give concrete and literal examples of questions and situations to aid understanding;
- Directly ask whether individuals understand, rather than expecting people to ask for clarification;
- Communicate using short and simple sentences, rather than complex words and long sentences.

Whenever possible, information about the research should be provided to each person on an individual, face-to-face basis. Careful consideration should be given to how relatives, carers and other members of the person's support network will be informed about the research, while ensuring that potential participants experience no coercion in making their decision whether or not to be involved in the research. The critical ethical issue is that people are involved without coercion. To assure other people that this has occurred, it is necessary to have a permanent record of the process of agreement. An audiotape of an oral discussion of the researcher and a participant involving information provision and decision-making can provide an even fuller record of the validity of the agreement obtained than a signature on a consent form.

Carers

Like service users, carers are a diverse group. Their views tend to differ from the interests of clinical research professionals, as well as the views of those they care for. Carers and service users can be interested in being involved in research for different reasons. Some people think that health research should have an emancipatory function, especially in terms of improving personal health or life opportunities. Carers may be more likely to see research as helping people with health problems or developing better services for people, and not necessarily as a personal emancipatory activity.

From the perspective of carers themselves, few accounts emerge of their personal reasons for becoming involved in research. For carers of people with disabilities, Brereton and Dawes (2003) suggest that the reasons include: an opportunity to be listened to and to feel valued, time to reflect on problems and a desire to help future carers. And, some of the negative risks of involvement are thought to include: the possibility of research evoking distress, taking up time, a concern by the disabled person that their privacy is being breached and difficulties in ending a supportive relationship with the researchers. This study focuses on 'new carers' of people who have experienced a stroke and suggested that carers might appreciate information, ongoing details about the study, attention to practicalities and briefing prior to any interviews. It touches on the benefits that carers may derive from participation but also the researcher's responsibilities around support. Other benefits to being engaged in research studies were outlined by Fine (2003) in relation to palliative care and in cancer care (Birchall et al. 2002), where carers and patients have been involved in research that has contributed to the development of standards of care. Yates et al. (1997) did not anticipate the benefit to carers of people with HIV of research involvement, yet found great potential for learning, sharing and support.

Challenges of involving carers in research include the following:

• Service user involvement has a longer history and is more advanced. Service user involvement appears to be intuitively easier to grasp, partly because it can be seen as a logical extension of good clinical practice.
• The majority of funding bodies require a commitment to involving service users in the research; fewer expect carer involvement.
• Identifying and contacting carers can be harder than contacting registered patients or service users.
• Carers may not have much time for involvement activities because of the full-time nature of their caring responsibilities. They may not be able to travel for meetings or spend days away.

- Consent of service users is often considered necessary in order that carers can be consulted or involved in research. However, some researchers and carers believe that carers should be involved in their own right.

In theory carers can be involved in all stages of research; however, some stages offer greater opportunities to contribute to decisions about the research. For example:

- Consulting carers on the topic of the research and developing an application for research funding
- Consulting carers on the methods of a research study and the detail of the questions to be asked
- Involving carers as advocates or representatives for a research study
- Involving carers in reviewing literature aimed at service users, carers or the public
- Assisting researchers to analyse and interpret the data
- Dissemination of the research findings to carers and those they care for

As with service user representation, carer 'representativeness' would require a large number of carefully selected carers who present the views of many carers (see 'Involvement' section). More realistically, enthusiastic and knowledgeable individual carers can be involved to provide 'a carer perspective'. There are benefits to involving more than one or two carers in any research study. It helps to show that carers can have multiple perspectives of the issues, rather than there being one 'carer view'. As research with foster carers shows, carers can learn from one another and identify what is important to them when they interact and 'share the insights that they alone can give into the difficulties and opportunities they experience' (Fleming 2005). In practical terms, inviting more than one carer to be involved can help to ensure that a carer perspective is represented throughout the research if a person is not able to attend or has to withdraw their involvement at any stage.

Carers can be accessed through voluntary sector organisations. For example:

- In the UK – Carers UK, Princess Royal Trust for Carers, Rethink (which specialises in working with carers and has local offices and carers centres)
- In the USA – Resources for Caregivers, Family Caregiver Alliance, National Family Caregivers Association, MUMS (Mothers United for Moral Support), Well Spouse Foundation
- Canada – Caregiver Network, Child and Family Canada
- Australia – Care Respite Centres, Carers Association (South Australia/Victoria), MOIRA Child and Family Support, Ozcarere (Australian Cancer Support and Resources)

People who join carers' centres and carers' groups usually have an awareness of themselves as being carers, but people who do not feel they would fit into the dominant 'carer' culture may in effect be excluded, for example it has only recently been widely recognised that there are many young carers. Specific health services, for example hospitals or early intervention teams may be useful for accessing friends, relatives, partners, siblings and so on, of people with health issues who do not see themselves as 'carers'.

Carers' ability to travel and spend many hours away from home is often limited as they are constrained by their caring obligations, lack of time, travel problems and so on. It is best to stipulate in advance how far and how often carers will need to travel and which expenses will be reimbursed, for example travel by public transport, standard class, and taxis, childcare, substitute care, meals, etc. by prior agreement only. Carers should be informed that they need to keep their receipts for reimbursement. As with the payment of service users, payment of fees to carers can be complicated because of social security benefit rules and organisational payroll systems (see Chapter 3, 'Payments' section). Consideration should always be given to a person's wishes about payment, impact on social security benefits, and the method of payment. Some carers prefer not to receive payment, but this should not be assumed.

Like service users, carers involved in research should be offered support for their additional responsibilities. In particular, specific types of research roles such as involvement in peer review or ethical committees require clear guidance and training about the role. Carers should be informed who will be providing support and what form this will take. Carers usually welcome opportunities to learn and to fulfil the role to the best of their ability if training is relevant to the role they are taking on – rather than being 'too general' research training or providing information that could be given in other ways. A practical solution can be to offer 'on the job' training, such as supervision and peer support meetings.

Key principles for practice

- There are many reasons and ways to bring a patient's viewpoint to all kinds of healthcare issues. Involving patients who are receiving health care in research requires striking a fine balance between the ethical duties of providing care and support, and achieving involvement that is accessible and meaningful.
- It is unethical to exclude people who are very sick from research if the correct safeguards and practical steps can be put in place so that they can be involved if they wish to participate.
- Patients with rare clinical conditions generally express great enthusiasm about improving care or services. Researchers need to be realistic and explain the scale and pace of improvements that can be made.
- Some people find it difficult to access mainstream health services and therefore to be involved in research. Researchers should be aware of potential barriers including disability, age, ethnicity, sexuality, people with severe learning disabilities and/or communication impairments, mental health problems, homelessness, substance abuse, geographical isolation, and refugee/asylum seeker status.
- Some people do not have the capacity to consent; however, the capacity to give informed consent is a continuum, and a person's capacity to make decisions may vary depending on the specific topic or area of life under consideration.
- Carers are a diverse group of people, who can bring their own perspectives to nursing and healthcare research. Their views tend to differ from the interests of clinical research professionals, as well as the views of those they care for.

References

Abma, T. (2005) Patient participation in health research: research with and for people with spinal cord injuries. *Qualitative Health Research,* 15 (10): 1310–28.

Addington-Hall, J. (2002) Research sensitivities to palliative care patients. *European Journal of Cancer Care,* 11 (3): 220–4.

Agrawal, M. (2003) Voluntariness in clinical research at the end of life. *Journal of Pain Symptom Management*, 25 (4): S25–32.

Bate, S. and Robert, G. (2007) *Bringing User Experience to Health Care Improvement: The Concepts, Methods and Practices of Experience-Based Design*. Oxford: Radcliffe Publishing.

Beresford, P. and Campbell, J. (1994) Disabled people, service users, user involvement and representation. *Disability & Society*, 9 (3): 315–325.

Birchall, M., Richardson, A., and Lee, L. (2002) Eliciting views of patients with head and neck cancer and carers on professionally derived standards for care. *British Medical Journal*, 324 (7336): 516–9.

Brereton, L. and Dawes, H. (2003) Building on carers' stories to enrich research. *Quality in Ageing*, 4 (4): 11–7.

Chadwick, R. (2001) Informed consent and genetic research. In: Doyal, L. and Tobias, J. (eds) *Informed Consent in Medical Research*, London: BMJ Books, pp. 203–10.

Cleary, P. (1999) The importance of patient surveys. *British Medical Journal*, 319: 720–1.

Cotterell, P., Clarke, P., Cowdrey, D., Kapp, J., Paine, M., and Wynn, D. (2005) *Influencing Palliative Care Project: A Participatory Study*. Worthing: Worthing and Southlands Hospitals NHS Trust.

Department of Health (2008) *Understanding What Matters: A Guide to Using Patient Feedback to Transform Care*. London: Department of Health.

Fine, P.G. (2003) Maximizing benefits and minimizing risks in palliative care research that involves patients near the end of life. *Journal of Pain & Symptom Management*, 25 (4): S53–62.

Fleming, J. (2005) Foster carers undertake research into birth family contact. In: Lowes, L. and Hulatt, I. (eds) *Involving Service Users in Health and Social Care Research*. London: Routledge.

Morgan, L., Fahs, P., and Klesh, J. (2005) Barriers to research participation identified by rural people. *Journal of Agricultural Safety & Health*, 11 (4): 407–14.

National Childbirth Trust (2001) *A Charter for Ethical Research in Maternity Care. Association for Improvements in Maternity Services*. London: The National Childbirth Trust.

Newman, E. and Kaloupek, D. (2004) The risks and benefits of participating in trauma focused research studies. *Journal of Traumatic Stress*, 17 (5): 383–94.

RCN (2005) *Informed Consent in Health and Social Care Research. Guidance for Nurses*. London: Royal College of Nursing.

Small, N. and Rhodes, P. (2000) *Too Ill to Talk? User Involvement and Palliative Care*. London: Routledge.

The Healthcare Commission (2006) *The Views of Hospital Inpatients in England: Key Findings from the 2006 Survey*. London: The Health Care Commission.

Williams, B. (1994) Patient satisfaction: A valid concept? *Social Science & Medicine*, 38: 509–16.

Wise, J. (2009) Part of hospitals' funding will depend on patient satisfaction ratings. *British Medical Journal*, 339: b5451.

Yates, B., McEwan, C., and Eadie, D. (1997) How to involve hard to reach groups: a consumer-led project with lay carers of people with advanced HIV infection. *Public Health*, 111 (5): 297–303.

Chapter 6

Involvement over the life course

Key summary points

- *Children and their parents*: Concerns about whether children and young people have the intellectual capacity or understanding to take a more active role in research often mean that parents are involved on their behalf. However, involving young people from the start of the research, not just as subjects of the research, can help to ensure that the topic is important to them and their families, as well as helping to identify any practical issues with the way the research is to be carried out.
- *School-age children*: Involving students in schools can avoid the risk of burdening sick children or those who are undergoing treatment or care. Schools can support access to different types of children and young people from different communities, age groups and backgrounds.
- *Young people*: Involving young people (12–21 year olds) in research can help to shape the way that research questions are constructed and the themes that the research should explore. They can offer a different perspective on what questions should be asked of respondents and the type of language that is used.
- *Adults*: There are times when research involves 'healthy' adult populations, for example to inform screening programmes, immunisation and health promotion work. In these research contexts researchers may need to consider reaching well adults through workplaces, higher education, social spaces, public spaces and using websites, media and press.
- *Older people*: The term older people covers a broad spectrum from the 'young old' to the 'old old', or in other words the Third Age of active leisure and personal fulfilment and the Fourth Age of greater dependence and degeneration. Access issues can be more of a problem for some older people because of mobility problems and fragility. Researchers need to carefully consider issues to do with ways of working and working environments as well as how best to communicate effectively with each person.

Children and their parents

Concerns about whether children and young people have the intellectual capacity or understanding to take a more active role in research often mean that they are often excluded or that parents are involved on their behalf. Like any other group of service

Handbook of Service User Involvement in Nursing and Healthcare Research, First Edition.
Elizabeth Morrow, Annette Boaz, Sally Brearley and Fiona Ross.
© 2012 Elizabeth Morrow, Annette Boaz, Sally Brearley and Fiona Ross.
Published 2012 by Blackwell Publishing Ltd.

users, children and young people can be involved in research as subjects or participants; indeed involvement is considered part of their human rights.

Parental representation can be at odds with the rights of the child to express their views freely in all matters affecting them (Article 12 of the United Nations Convention 1989). Human rights place a duty on the government and public services and their constituent agencies, to treat all individuals with fairness, equality, dignity and respect (Hart 1992). However, children and young people are often not informed about their rights or how to take action if their rights have been violated (Willow 1999). A guide produced by the National Children's Bureau (Young 2008) offers children and young people the opportunity to become more familiar with the Human Rights Act 1998 and other human rights legislation.

Of course, the law and good practice still applies to the involvement of children in research. A report by Dimond (2002) summarises the law concerning research with children, consent, parental consent and risks to the child. The Royal College of Paediatrics and Child Health Ethics Advisory Committee has produced guidelines for the ethical conduct of medical research involving children. A review by O'Quigley (2000) on listening to children draws from published research about legal, administrative and mediatory processes, as well as children's views on how they would like to be involved. The report outlines some successful ways of listening to children:

- If possible, children should be assured of confidentiality; if this is not possible then the limits to confidentiality should be made clear at the outset.
- Adults should be aware of developmental and cultural factors but should beware of making assumptions about the individual child on the basis of these.
- Adults should adopt a non-intrusive style of interviewing with the aim of learning from the child.
- The child needs adequate information in order to express views.
- Questions should be simple and direct; indirect questions should be avoided as these are experienced by children as 'trick' questions.
- Adults should be open-minded and non-judgemental, and allow the child to raise their agendas and not simply respond to the adult agenda.
- Adults should allow the child to tell the whole of their story, without interrupting or rushing to interpretation.
- Younger children may prefer to speak if they have a friend with them.
- Good communication is more likely to occur if adults see children's abilities and competencies as being *different* from rather than *lesser* than adults'.
- Some children may not want to participate in decision-making at all.
- The interviewer should be alert for any sign of distress in the child and acknowledge it.

Dixon-Woods et al. (1999) describe the debates about entering into more active research partnerships with children and argue that evaluation of outcomes of involvement needs encouragement from government bodies together with promotion of quality information to reassure parents that this will not lead to adverse effects in the long-term. A key point of the following case study (Box 6.1) is that involving young people from the start of the research, not just as subjects of the research, can help to ensure that the

Box 6.1   National Institute for Health Research (NIHR) Medicines for Children Research Network (MCRN)

Case study

Jennifer Newman

My name is Jenny Newman. I am the Consumer Liaison Officer for the NIHR Medicines for Children Research Network. We are a national network and the Coordinating Centre is based at the Institute of Child Health in Liverpool. My main role is to involve parents, carers and, more importantly, children and young people in the networks' activities.

Issue/scenario: 'Involving children'

In 2006 we set up a pilot young people's group to explore how young people could be involved in MCRN activities and have their say in the design of clinical research. The pilot was such a success that the group has now been re-launched to involve more children and young people. Furthermore, four additional groups have been established to form one large national young person's advisory group. These groups are based in four MCRN Local Research Networks (LRNs): Trent, West Midlands, London and Bristol. Each group comprises of approximately 10–17 young members, between 8 and 19 years that have experience of living with a childhood condition, illness, disability or taking medicines. A training programme for each group is now running, covering research methods and clinical research. To date, group members have been involved in a wide range of activities, including helping researchers with their projects, working with organisations such as the Medicines and Healthcare products Regulatory Agency (MHRA) and the National Research Ethics Service (NRES). During 2010–2011 the group will continue to work with researchers and various organisations as well as advising other young people what researchers are finding out (through summaries and a website which the groups will develop), present at MCRN related conferences to highlight the work of the young persons' group and carry out their own mini research project.

Key issues to be aware of:

- Involving young people from the start of the research, not just as subjects of the research can help to identify whether the topic is important to them and their families, and whether there are any important practical aspects or issues that have been overlooked.
- Existing groups and networks like ours can be a useful starting point for getting advice and information. It may not always be possible or appropriate to set up your own young people's group if there is little time or resources to do so.
- Most information for children has been adapted from adult information; it is often too long, and uses complex medical or legal terminology. Children and young people need accessible information about what they are being asked to do in the research and what they can expect to happen.

Solution/helpful ideas:

- The young people's group have produced guidance for researchers about the design and content of patient information leaflets specifically for young people. This can be accessed on our website (www.mcrn.org.uk).
- It can be helpful to plan to work with young people to identify ethical issues that might arise with consent processes or information giving during medicines research. An established group like the Medicines for Children Research Network can provide comments or feedback on proposed research if sufficient time is set aside before ethical approval for the research is sought.

> ➤ **Introduce yourself:** Be sensitive to local concerns about children, for example parental fears or worries about professional intervention in family life.
>
> ➤ **Respect children's views and feelings:** Emphasise that you are interested in children's descriptions in their own words and that there are no right or wrong answers. They can leave an activity if they don't want to carry on. They don't have to answer all the questions or participate in all the activities. Be respectful that a child may be reluctant to speak about a sensitive topic.
>
> ➤ **Your conduct:** Be punctual, organised and listen. Keep appointments. Find the room, set out chairs and materials in advance. Turn off your mobile phone. Offer refreshments. Keep a flexible timetable and be prepared to have a break between activities.

Figure 6.1   Key ideas for involving children.

topic is important to them and their families, as well as helping to identify any practical issues with the way the research is to be carried out.

There is some good practice in involving children and young people in research but there is also scope for development. A review by Clark et al. (2003) demonstrates that some imaginative methods are being used by researchers, practitioners and consultants to listen to and to consult with young children. These include methods adapted from work with older children such as interviews, questionnaires, group work and participatory games. Other techniques such as observation have been combined with the use of media, role play, drawing and puppets. Key ideas for working with children are presented in Figure 6.1. In some areas of health service development children are being provided with the opportunity to be involved directly in issues affecting them, such as decisions about the design of hospitals for children and young people or the development of health information websites. Researchers need to be careful not to raise expectations about the type of broader health information or interventions that can be provided as a result of the research (Clark et al. 2001).

Alderson and Morrow (2004) examine the ethical issues of social research projects, which consult with children and young people from the planning stages through to the reporting and dissemination stages. They suggest that involving children in research requires the building of trusting relationships with families and children over time. Not all children and families will perceive research in the same way, and certain groups may need more support and information than others to be involved (see Chapter 7). Researchers must retain a clear focus on ethical questions to address the concerns that may be raised by parents, children and others and to respect parents' responsibilities for their children. This needs to be a two-way learning process where researchers gain an understanding of

> ➢ It is best practice to obtain informed consent from children, their parents or carriers, and community members.
>
> ➢ To do this you must explain:
> (a) who you are
> (b) what will happen to any personal or private information gained
> (c) the details of the research and involvement
> (d) any agreement to anonymity and confidentiality
> (e) procedure for breach of confidentiality/child protection.
>
> ➢ Ask children for permission to audio record, take photos or video them, and explain why.

Figure 6.2   Key ideas for informed consent with children.

> ➢ At the end of your visit/the meeting, explain to the children what will happen next with the information they have provided.
>
> ➢ Ask if anyone has any questions.
>
> ➢ Allow time for the children to prepare questions before you leave.
>
> ➢ Thank the children for their involvement.
>
> ➢ Let them know who to speak to if they have any questions or concerns afterwards.

Figure 6.3   Key ideas for ending involvement with children.

their expectations and concerns, alongside the formalities of gaining informed consent. Key ideas for informed consent with children are presented in Figure 6.2. It is also important to give consideration to how involvement will be ended; see Figure 6.3 for some ideas.

School-age children

One way of gaining views from young people is through schools. There are a number of benefits of involving schools in research including:

• Involving students in schools can avoid the risk of burdening sick children or those who are undergoing treatment or care.

Box 6.2   Engagement in 'safe places' with school-age children and young people

Case study

Professor Jane Coad

I am a Professor in Children and Family Nursing, based at Coventry University. My research interests are involving children and young people in the development of health services using participatory arts-based methods.

Interviews with children and young people about hospital design

We undertook a project to ascertain views of school-aged children and young people across a broad range of ages and abilities about design preferences for a purpose-built Children's Unit in a new hospital (1, 2). Full ethical approval was given by the Local Research Ethics Committee for the project but we also assigned an adult gatekeeper – a Senior Play Therapist who was not an active researcher for the project. From the outset in order to gain consent without coercion we had agreement for participants to be involved in the study.

The study comprised of two phases. Phase 1 consisted of semi-structured interviews and phase 2 consisted of questionnaires posted to a 6-month retrospective sample. Children and young people (aged 10–16) also acted as an 'expert group' to the project and informed the project at all stages. In phase 1 it was important to create 'safe places' for engagement; 60 arts-based one-to-one interviews were conducted with school-aged children and young people aged from 8 to 18 years in the 'old' hospital setting including ten children and young people with learning difficulties and physical impairments. Settings included the children's ward, the bedside and outpatient departments whilst children and their families were waiting for appointments. Ensuring privacy during the interview in a busy hospital environment gave us many challenges but we only used 'spaces' such as the playroom on the ward, private rooms if the interviews were by the bedside, and a free room when in the outpatient department.

We also needed space around us for the interview as children and young people were invited to undertake drawings and were offered a range of textile/design materials to help them describe their preferences for the new hospital ward environment. One challenge was getting a consensus on colour from the 'child's perspective'. The children and young people's 'expert group' gave us the idea of using paint colour charts (like for home-based decorating). Consequently, each participant was asked about their colour preferences in the relevant areas of the new hospital using specifically devised colour design charts. These included a range of over 100 colours, so subtlety of colours like bold and/or pastels could be viewed and chosen. Each colour was printed as a thick line, which was subsequently scored as 1 to 9 in the predetermined colour spectrum (starting at 1 in the left-hand corner, as the *most pale,* to 9 in the right-hand corner, being the *most dark*). The same tool was used for each participant's choice recorded using a tape recorder.

We felt that using such an approach ensured that children and young people could tell us their likes and dislikes in a way that was fun, meaningful and where they felt safe. Most notable findings included strong preferences for colour. It was 'expected' that the children and young people might choose the brighter colours on the selection colour charts offered, but without any prompts children and young people repeatedly choose paler and mid-colours with blue-green colours being the most popular. Hospital designers responded by decorating the new Children's Unit according to the children and young people's preferences.

Key issues:

• The additional burden of research on sick children/inpatients and families can be difficult at times.

- What researchers may think of as basic concepts may be too difficult for the child or young person to understand. Some words may have a very particular meaning so it is important to check the individual's level of language and understanding.
- Safe spaces which are places where children and young people feel safe and comfortable should be provided even if the space is very public. The case study highlights how we overcame this.
- Children and young people may find it difficult to relate to unfamiliar people, such as members of the research team. It can also be difficult to establish trust in the context of a one-off interview.

Helpful ideas:

- All researchers on the team need to have appropriate skills to work with children and young people, such as an ability to express ideas simply. Researchers should be flexible in following the children and young people's lead in the discussion and listen carefully to their use of words.
- Where possible involve existing groups of children and young people who know each other already. If this is not possible, create social and play contexts that facilitate easy and relaxed communication. Provide fun art materials, snacks or drinks (if allowed), relaxed seating arrangements and child-friendly rooms.

(1) Coad, J., Coad, N. et al. (2008) Children and young people's preference of thematic design and colour for their hospital environment. *British Journal of Child Health*, March, 33–48.
(2) Coad, J. and Evans, R. (2008) Children and young people's engagement in the data analysis process. A practical framework. *Children and Society*, January, 2, 41–52.

- Schools can support access to different types of children and young people from different communities, age groups and backgrounds.
- Students may feel more relaxed and able to talk about health issues if they are amongst peers – but the opposite can also be true depending on the topic of the research.
- Students and parents may be more open to research if researchers take time to work with young people and their teachers in schools.
- As well as lending support to the research, teachers can provide their views and input into the research.
- Schools can provide meeting spaces that are generally safer and more suited to young people than other social spaces.

Schools are often approached by researchers as part of promoting health research and gaining community support for research work. For example, the Health Research for Schools team in the Department of Health Sciences of the University of Leicester was formed to promote communication with the local community about health research. The aim is to work with children in schools to explain what health research is, and why it is important. Whilst this type of activity is not classifiable as involvement, it supports more active forms of involvement by informing teachers, parents and young people about health research and encouraging closer links between professional researchers and school pupils. For researchers involving schools in research can be beneficial for gaining a sense of advocacy that the research is legitimate and important to the health or well-being of young people (see Box 6.2).

Young people

In the UK, the term 'young people' is generally used to mean those who are between 12 and 21 years of age. A guide to actively involving young people in research has been produced by INVOLVE (2004) to give researchers and commissioners of research guidance about when and how to involve young people. The guide looks at the issues of involving young researchers and ways of supporting young people's involvement. It particularly highlights the importance of involving young people in deciding how they will be involved to ensure their participation is not tokenistic or manipulated by adults.

The Triumph and Success Project (France 2000) recruited eight young people aged between 15 and 21 from different social and economic backgrounds to help undertake research on youth transitions in Sheffield. The research project was run by a team of youth workers and supported by professional researchers from a local university. Young researchers were involved in designing questionnaires and undertook a survey with nearly 750 young people and face-to-face interviews with 60 young people from a range of backgrounds across Sheffield. They also helped to make the language of the research more 'youth-friendly' and to encourage active participation of diverse youth groups in the research process. The evaluation of Triumph and Success found that when it comes to engaging young people and keeping them involved, the following are important:

- Having a well-defined, systematic recruitment strategy in place prior to initiation
- Having both wide advertising and a targeted approach that focuses on 'hard to reach' young people which will help recruit a diverse group of participants
- Having a recruitment process that gives young people details about what the work will entail and the level of commitment that is expected of them
- Allowing young people to choose to be involved
- Giving serious consideration to the diversity and representativeness of the group of young people involved
- Creating a participation structure that allows young people to leave and return to the project when they feel ready
- Encouraging and developing support networks within the group of young people involved
- Having a coordinator that can motivate, drive and support diverse groups of young people
- Having a youth work support structure that is responsive to young people's needs
- Having fun!

The evaluation also found that while the level of influence young people can have on the research process can be high, it may be limited because they are generally involved after the questions to be investigated have been selected (France 2000). It is likely that young people can have a greater influence if they are involved earlier on in the process. Another issue is that young people's exit from the research can be difficult if there is no clear strategy for ending and moving on.

Clark et al. (2001) have looked at different methods of involving different groups of young people in different aspects of the research process and on different issues.

Box 6.3   A young person's view of VIK (Very Important Kid) panel

Case Study

Amy Feltham

My name is Amy. I am 16 years old and I work as a nursery assistant. In my spare time I am part of the VIK panel at YoungMinds (www.youngminds.org.uk).

YoungMinds VIK panel

The VIK panel looks at important issues in the mental health system. We campaign for better rights for young people with mental illness. There are about 22 young people on the panel, who meet every 6 weeks. There is a regional officer and two representatives from each region. I represent the London region.

At our meetings we spend a full day doing activities. It is a good way to meet other young people who I can talk to without having to explain all the mental health jargon. The regional officers are there on meeting days, as well as Rosie, who sets up the VIK days.

What makes it work?

When we meet it is clear to everyone that if we don't want to do a certain activity during the day that's fine, we can do something else, or sit out in a separate room. If there is part of the day I don't like I can tell my regional officer, Erin, and she can help me to leave the activity without feeling embarrassed. The flexible approach that YoungMinds use with us is really good – like letting me re-number things if the current numbering is making me anxious. It really does make a difference.

Young people facilitators help to organise the meetings, as well as participating in the activities. They know how it feels to participate in the days, so can help plan the activities and the structure of the day to suit everyone. They also help to make sure that the little considerations are thought about, like having decaffeinated drinks and making sure that everyone's dietary needs are taken care of.

Most of the activities are run in small groups of five or six young people, where we discuss specific areas. It is good to be in a group because we can bounce ideas off each other and other people can help me put things into the right words. It's really good to know that other people are thinking the same thing and that we can find ways to do something about it. Some of the recent topics we have discussed are how policies and procedures need to change in schools and what should be included in training days – it all adds towards helping young people with mental health issues. Sometimes we talk about our personal stories and it helps illustrate the point better, but there is no pressure to do this. YoungMinds keeps a file about each of us with emails and information in it, but we know we can ask to read the file at any time. We also have 'ground rules' for the meetings, like 'what is said in the room stays in the room', and these apply to the staff and the young people. The easier it is to trust everyone at YoungMinds, the easier it is to talk about different issues.

Having mental health issues has been a very negative experience for me. Being part of the VIK panel means I can make something positive out of it. I know I am helping to change some of the bad things about the mental health system. YoungMinds give us email feedback about what is happening so that we know when we have helped to make things change for the better.

Key issues to be aware of:

• Getting the little things right helps make sure the big things run smoothly.
• Trust is a big issue, especially confidentiality and knowing what is being said about you.
• Mental health can be a very negative experience and being part of a group like the VIK panel can help turn bad experiences in to positive changes.

Helpful ideas:

- Researchers should find out more about groups like YoungMinds, because they have loads of good ideas and know how to work with young people.
- When researchers ask a young person a question they should listen to the response – not just presume they know the answer.

It can be helpful to involve young people through local or national youth organisations to gain their backing and support for working with young people, as illustrated by the following case study (Box 6.3). A useful report by Kirby (1999) is based on participatory research done within Save the Children and other organisations, and includes case study examples. It explores the ways in which young people can participate in the different stages of the research process and some of the ethical issues. Other research has focused on issues of involving young people with learning disabilities or mental health problems in research (Claveirole 2004, Centre for Research on Families and Relationships 2005).

Adults

As discussed in Chapter 2, the meaning of involving 'service users' in research is wider than those patients who are currently receiving treatment or care. In some research contexts it may also include those who consider themselves healthy and well and those who have no current need for health care. Although nursing and healthcare research are generally concerned with the experience of illness or service use, there are times when the research involves healthy adult populations, for example research to inform health screening programmes, immunisation and health promotion work.

Involving well adults in research can be difficult because of defining a representative sample, and because individuals may not see themselves as having anything to say about nursing or health care. There can also be practical issues of reaching healthy adults, for example they are likely to be at work at times when there are opportunities to be involved in research. Adults may also have child care or other caring responsibilities outside of working hours that prevent them being involved in research.

Ways of reaching well adults include:

- Workplaces: for example, through occupational health or health and safety groups
- Higher education: for example, university student unions or courses
- Social spaces: for example, meeting with members of societies or faith groups
- Public spaces: for example, shopping centres or outside of football grounds
- Web-based: for example, websites, online surveys, online social networks
- Media: using local radio or television for advertising
- Press: news articles in newspapers or magazines

Older people

Assumptions are often made that involving older people in research is difficult. These assumptions hinge around concerns that health problems and mental capacity may intervene with participation and understanding, for example age-related degenerative mental health problems may have implications for understanding and consent. However, generally there is a good record of older people, and veterans, being involved in health and social care research, possibly because they have more time to participate or more interest in health and social care issues as users of these services (Boaz and Hayden 2002). It is also important to recognise that the term older people covers a broad spectrum from the 'young old' to the 'old old', or in other words the Third Age of active leisure and personal fulfilment and the Fourth Age of greater dependence and degeneration.

A review of the literature (Fudge et al. 2007) shows that benefits to older people of participating in research include increased knowledge, awareness and confidence, meeting others in similar situations, and empowering older people to become active in their community regarding decisions/policies which affect them. Common barriers to involving older people include cultural divisions, language barriers, research skills capacity, ill health, time and resources. One of the key benefits of involvement emphasised by older women involved in The Older Women's Lives and Voices project was the breaking down of isolation: understanding that they were not alone and that others were going through the same experiences of growing older (Warren and Cook 2005).

Older people tend to inhabit different social spaces to those outlined in the previous section, which has implications for recruitment and methods of involvement. Involvement of older people can be successful if researchers 'outreach' to social and public spaces. As with children, reaching out beyond healthcare settings can avoid the risk of burdening those who are sick or who are undergoing treatment or care. Older people may be members of local societies or faith groups through which they may be able to give their time to be involved in nursing and healthcare research.

Access issues can be more of a problem for older people because of mobility problems and fragility. There is evidence that if methods of involvement are right, attrition of older people from research is not a problem (Carter et al. 1991; Ross et al. 2005). Researchers need to carefully consider issues to do with ways of working and working environments, such as how to support older people as research advisors (Tozer and Thornton 1995). For example, due to the greater likelihood of hearing and sight problems in older people it is essential to spend time planning in advance how best to communicate effectively with each person (see Chapter 7). A related point is that older people are less likely to make use of web-based information and communication, but this is changing. If these methods are selected researchers are likely to need to offer training and support.

Frail older people have been relatively neglected in the growth of consultation and service user involvement (Barnes and Bennett 1998). An obvious hurdle has been the relative difficulty of involving frail people, many of whom may not venture readily from home, in service users' groups within academic settings. Reed et al. (2004) describe partnerships with older people as taking place against a background of academic research traditions and norms which can present obstacles to collaboration. Whether or not this is always the case, older people can sometimes hold different values about health care than other sectors of the general population. For example, their expectations about the use of public funds can mean that it is necessary to discuss personal preferences for payments for being involved in research (see Chapter 3).

Key principles for practice

- As with other groups of service users, involving young people from the start of the research, not just as subjects of the research, can help to ensure that the topic is important to them and their families, as well as helping to identify any practical issues with the way the research is to be carried out.
- Where possible avoid the risk of burdening sick people or those who are undergoing treatment or care by 'reaching out' to service users in other types of social and public spaces, such as schools and faith groups.
- Service users from different generations can offer a different perspective on what questions should be asked of respondents and the type of language that is used.
- In situations where research involves 'healthy' adult populations researchers should consider reaching well adults through workplaces, higher education, social spaces, public spaces and using websites, media and press.
- When working with older people researchers need to be especially careful to consider issues to do with ways of working and working environments as well as how best to communicate effectively with each person.

References

Alderson, P. and Morrow, V. (2004) *Ethics, Social Research and Consulting with Children and Young People*. Barkingside: Barnardo's.

Article 12 of the United Nations Convention (1989) *The UN Convention on the Rights of the Child*.

Barnes, M. and Bennett, G. (1998) Frail bodies, courageous voices: older people influencing community care. *Health and Social Care in the Community,* 6: 102–111.

Boaz, A. and Hayden, C. (2002) Pro-active evaluators: Enabling research to be useful, usable and used. *Evaluation*, 8 (4): 440–453.

Carter, W., Elward, K., Malmgren, J., Martin, M., and Larson, E. (1991) Participation of older adults in health programs and research: a critical review of the literature. *The Gerontologist*, 31 (5): 584–92.

Centre for Research on Families and Relationships (2005) Centre for Research on Families and Relationships (accessible at http://www.crfr.ac.uk/).

Clark, J., Dyson, A., Meagher, N., Robson, E., and Wooten, M. (eds) (2001) *Young People as Researchers: Possibilities, Problems and Politics*. Leicester: National Youth Agency.

Clark, A., McQuail, S., and Moss, P. (2003) Exploring the field of listening to and consulting with young children. Department of Education and Skills. Research report No. 445, 2003.

Claveirole, A. (2004) Listening to young voices: challenges of research with adolescent mental health service users. *Journal of Psychiatric & Mental Health Nursing*, 11: 253–60.

Dimond, B. (2002) Step 45: research 5: children. *British Journal of Midwifery*, 10 (9): 573.

Dixon-Woods, M., Young, B., and Heney, D. (1999) Partnerships with children. *British Medical Journal*, 319: 778–80.

Fudge, N., Wolfe, C., and McKevitt, C. (2007) Involving older people in health research. *Age & Ageing*, 36 (5): 492–500.

France, A. (2000) *Youth Researching Youth: The Triumph and Success Research Project*. York: Joseph Rowntree Foundation, 2000.

Hart, D. (1992) *An Introduction to Children's Rights*. London: National Children's Bureau.

INVOLVE (2004) A guide to actively involving young people in research: for researchers, research commissioners and managers. (Available from http://www.invo.org.uk/)

Kirby, P. (1999) *Involving Young Researchers: How to Enable Young People to Design and Conduct Research*. York: Joseph Rowntree Foundation.

O'Quigley, A. (2000) *Listening to Children's Views. The Findings and Recommendations of Recent Research*. York: Joseph Rowntree Foundation.

Reed, J., Weiner, R., and Cook, G. (2004) Partnership research with older people – moving towards making the rhetoric a reality. *Journal of Clinical Nursing,* 13 (3a): 3–10.

Ross, F., Donovan, S., Brearley, S., Victor, C., Cottee, M., Crowther, P., and Clark, E. (2005) Involving older people in research: methodological issues. *Health & Social Care in the Community,* 13 (3): 268–75.

Tozer, R. and Thornton, P. (1995) *A Meeting of Minds: Older People as Research Advisors*. York: Social Policy Research Unit, University of York.

Warren, L. and Cook, J. (2005) Working with older women in research. In: Lowes, L. and Hulatt, I. (eds) *Involving Service Users in Health and Social Care Research*. London: Routledge.

Willow, C. (1999) *It's Not Fair: Young People's Reflections on Children's Rights*. London: Children's Society.

Young, J. (2008) *Human Rights Are Children's Rights*. London: National Children's Bureau.

Chapter 7

Seldom-heard groups

Key summary points

- *Involving seldom-heard groups*: People within seldom-heard groups may find it difficult to access services and are less likely to be heard by service professionals and decision-makers. Multiple barriers and circumstances affect seldom-heard groups including lack of awareness, communication barriers and access issues.
- *People with physical disabilities*: Access is likely to be more of an issue for some people with physical disabilities and this means paying careful attention to individual needs and working environments prior to involvement.
- *The deaf and people who are hard of hearing*: Different groups of people with hearing difficulties tend to have different characteristics and types of communication preferences. Researchers need to consider using a range of ways of communicating including lip-reading, sign language, and large screen projection of speech-to-text.
- *People who are blind or partially sighted*: As with other seldom-heard groups, the methods of a research study may need to be refined to capture the diversity of strengths and needs of blind or partially sighted people. Researchers therefore need to be aware of adequately costing for additional resources and time required for recruitment, providing multimedia forms of information, and for researcher visual awareness training.
- *People with learning disabilities*: Working with people who have learning disabilities requires finding ways to effectively communicate with each service user, their carers and family members. Individualised communication involves using personal vocabularies, along with signs, graphic symbols and photographs to supplement spoken language.
- *People with degenerative cognitive impairment*: Involving people with cognitive impairment in research raises issues about the ethics of involvement, consent, communication and the impact of involvement. However, these seldom-heard groups can be involved in research if methods are tailored to their circumstances.
- *People with mental health problems*: Mental health service users are a seldom-heard group but there is a strong tradition of involvement in this field and good evidence to show that they can be successfully involved as employees, trainers, or researchers in the evaluation and development of services.

Handbook of Service User Involvement in Nursing and Healthcare Research, First Edition.
Elizabeth Morrow, Annette Boaz, Sally Brearley and Fiona Ross.
© 2012 Elizabeth Morrow, Annette Boaz, Sally Brearley and Fiona Ross.
Published 2012 by Blackwell Publishing Ltd.

> • *Black and minority ethnic groups*: BME groups are seldom-heard because they may suffer racism, health inequalities and language barriers as well as more subtle issues of professionals' cultural ignorance and lack of awareness of BME issues.

Involving seldom-heard groups

The term 'seldom-heard groups' is sometimes used to mean under-represented people who use or might potentially use health services and who are less likely to be heard by service professionals and decision-makers. It includes people who find it difficult to access services (see Chapter 5, 'Carers' Section). Such groups may also be referred to as 'marginalized' or 'vulnerable', though these terms can mean different things in different contexts, and some people may not wish to be described in these terms (Steel 2005).

Multiple barriers and circumstances affect seldom-heard groups. Many people in seldom-heard groups struggle to fulfil their basic life needs, which can limit the extent to which they have time to be involved in nursing or healthcare research. It is also likely that people within seldom-heard groups have a lack of awareness of research or a suspicion of professional researchers. Some seldom-heard groups can experience language barriers, societal discrimination and feelings of isolation from the rest of the community. They may also find it difficult to access information and/or culturally appropriate resources to help them understand what is available to them. For these reasons seldom-heard groups may find it difficult to engage with healthcare professionals and researchers, especially if their interactions with health services are episodic and they have transient lifestyles.

Issues of communication can act as barriers to involvement of seldom-heard groups in research, for example:

• There may not be enough thinking time in research project timeframes for some people with communication impairments.
• The language used in research can be technical and different terms might be used than in everyday language.
• Communication may be too fast, or incompatible with some communication methods.
• Computer-based communication can exclude some seldom-heard groups.

In addition, there may be practical barriers such as

• Lack of accessible transport or funding for transportation
• Lack of information about involvement, purpose and what might be achieved
• Noisy environments which make communication difficult
• Written information that is too long and complicated
• Difficult group dynamics or relationships between different groups of people, dominating persons or failure to respect other people's perspectives
• Lack of understanding about different people's roles and expectations for involvement

Researchers from the Social Care Institute for Excellence (SCIE 2008) have suggested several key ways to address barriers to involving seldom-heard groups:

- Treating people with respect and valuing individual contributions
- Providing clear and supportive communication
- Describing clearly what someone can expect from getting involved and what they are expected to contribute
- Making sure people know they can say 'no' to getting involved
- Offering a variety of activities and ways to get involved, such as helping others, learning and socialising

The following case study (Box 7.1) provides insight into how the idea of being involved in research can be overwhelming, even for experienced healthcare professionals. Embracing the patient voice can take time but involvement in research can help a person come to terms with having an illness or undergoing treatment.

People with physical disabilities

Involving people with physical disabilities right from the beginning can help to confirm that the research is worth doing and that it will be feasible to use particular approaches and methods. A good resource to begin with when planning to involve people with disabilities in research is to make use of disability directories to identify and link with established organisations. Some examples are listed below.

- In the UK: Ability, Directory of UK Self Help Groups and Support Organisations, Focus on disability
- In USA: Abilityinfo (Disability Information for Students and Professionals), American Disability Association, Disability Resources, Disabled People International
- Canada: Ability on Line Toronto, Canadian Abilities Foundation
- Australia: Challenge Disability Services, DIAL (Disability Information Network of Australia), DICE (Disability Information and Communication Exchange NSW), DIRSCA (Disability Information in South Australia)
- New Zealand: Disability Information Service, Disabled Persons Assembly

An individual person's disabilities may be congenital – meaning the person was born with the condition – or a result of injury, muscular dystrophy, multiple sclerosis, cerebral palsy, amputation, heart disease, pulmonary disease or another health condition. Some persons may have non-visible disabilities which include pulmonary disease, respiratory disorders, epilepsy and other limiting conditions.

Access is likely to be more of an issue for people with mobility impairment and this means paying careful attention to working environments (see Chapter 4) when involving people with arthritis, cerebral palsy, multiple sclerosis, muscular dystrophy, paralysis, Parkinson's Disease or stroke. One of the major difficulties persons with physical disabilities can face is gaining access to buildings, rooms and other facilities. However, as with any other group of service users, researchers should not presume to know what any individual person needs to enable them to be involved. Personal access requirements should be discussed with each person in confidence prior to their

Box 7.1 Embracing the patient/carer voice

Case study

Julie Wray, Researcher/Healthcare Professional/Survivor

I trained as a nurse and then a midwife in the late 1970s and early 1980s. I have practised in the USA and in many parts of the UK, covering hospital and community care settings. As a clinical practitioner I have always been taught to put the patient at the heart of everything and show a caring attitude at all times. I feel that I benefited from some excellent role models and nurses who inspired me to be the best and have high standards towards caring and compassion. As a research-minded nurse academic I have led numerous research studies focused upon patient experience of care. I believe strongly in embracing the patient/carer voice and in caring for the person, not the illness. After my own experience of cancer I have promoted complementary therapies and a positive approach to help others. I keep a blog to share my views and thoughts on breast cancer and some tips to inspire. (http://myvoiceandbreastcancer.blogspot.com/)

Issue/Scenario:

I was diagnosed with breast cancer in 2006. I was absolutely livid and angry; it was such a shock as I had no risk factors at all and only attended the 'one-stop' clinic as a precaution. Within a matter of minutes my life changed completely. I was busy at work, writing up my PhD and planning a fantastic holiday to Italy with my sons and husband – no time to be ill! But within a matter of days I had surgery, followed by chemotherapy, more surgery and then radiotherapy. Almost 12 months in treatment with plenty hospital appointments and contacts with healthcare professionals: such exposure provides huge insights into the NHS and the people who work in the caring professions.

I have to say from the very outset I was invited to participate in research studies. At first I found this annoying as my capacity to concentrate on what was happening was such that considering the details of research studies was too overwhelming; so at first I refused. Later on I agreed to be in a study – one that was focused on the experiences of newly diagnosed patients and their carer/s. I mention this as it was my contact and talks with the research nurse that I valued highly. As we talked about all my concerns she was thoughtful, caring, compassionate and informative. Other staff I met displayed caring and kindness. I met amazing nurses and doctors. I admit that I was assertive and as a nurse I had insider knowledge about the NHS. That said though I can reveal that I only came across one nurse who was inappropriate and lacked sensitivity, she implied that my cancer was very advanced and a rare form – in my mind she stepped too far over the professional boundary and left me devastated. I later found out that this information was not true. Why I mention this is that I managed this incident by asking that she had no part to play in my care and my request was respected and I have no contact. I now have lymphoedema which annoys me but again I have come to terms with it. I joined the breast cancer care service user partnership in 2009, as I feel passionate about listening to service user experience and research on survivorship.

Key issues to be aware of:

- Service users generally have much to offer, but the illness can be enough to deal with and the idea of being involved in research can seem overwhelming.
- One common problem/issue is that it takes time to be well again.
- An issue that I faced was dealing with anger about having got cancer.

Solution/helpful ideas:

- I have found that accepting my treatment alongside complementary therapies and yoga really helped.
- One solution for us has been to have fun, enjoy the moment, and give yourself a treat often.
- It can be helpful to talk with people you know or professionals that you trust or access breast cancer websites and join one of their discussion forums or go for long walks!

involvement. It is also better to plan to hold meetings or other research events in localities and buildings that support inclusive access.

The deaf and people who are hard of hearing

People with hearing difficulties identify themselves in different ways, but there are four main categories:

- Hard of hearing
- Deafened
- Deaf
- Deafblind

These different groups tend to have different characteristics and types of communication preferences. People who describe themselves as hard of hearing are likely to be older people (but not necessarily so), they probably have had a gradual loss of hearing, are likely to have some hearing, may wear a hearing aid for all or part of the time, are likely to use speech, lip-reading and the written word, and may have tinnitus (noises in the ear).

People who describe themselves as deafened are likely to have become deaf after fully hearing, are likely to have a severe or total hearing loss, are likely to use speech, lip-reading and the written word, they may have tinnitus, are unlikely to benefit from wearing a hearing aid, and may have a cochlear implant.

People who describe themselves as deaf (sign language users) are proud to see themselves as part of a deaf community, have probably been deaf since birth or early childhood, may have gone to a school for deaf children, may not use speech to communicate, probably use sign language, consider themselves to be part of a linguistic minority. Some hearing people can be seen as part of the deaf community. These are likely to be hearing people that use sign language, brothers and sisters of deaf people, or the hearing children of deaf parents.

People who describe themselves as deafblind may have differing degrees and causes of sight and hearing loss, may use speech and hearing aids, may use Braille or large print, or amplified audio tapes, may use a manual alphabet, or block letters written on the hand, may use sign language, may carry a red and white stick. Figure 7.1 illustrates some key ideas for communicating with someone who is deaf or hard of hearing. Sign language interpreters interpret from one language to another. In the UK this is usually from British sign language (BSL) to spoken or written English, or spoken or written English to BSL, but in different countries different forms of sign language are used. Sign languages are as diverse as spoken languages and can also have regional variations. Deaf people in different countries do not use the same sign language, but some sign languages do have a similar structure.

At conferences and larger meetings, written information can be projected on to a big screen or on to smaller screens around the room. Speech-to-text reporting is suitable for deaf people who are comfortable reading English, often at high speed and sometimes for up to a couple of hours at a time. Speech-to-text reporters use systems called Palantype® or Stenograph®. They use a special keyboard to type every word that is spoken by a

> ➤ Make sure you have face-to-face or eye-to-eye contact with the person you are talking to.
> ➤ Find a suitable place to talk, with good lighting and away from noise and distractions.
> ➤ Even if someone is wearing a hearing aid they may also need to lip-read.
> ➤ If you are using communication support always remember to talk directly to the person you are communicating with, not the interpreter.
> ➤ Speak clearly but not too slowly, and don't exaggerate your lip movements.
> ➤ Use natural facial expressions and gestures.
> ➤ If you're talking to a deaf person and a hearing person, don't just focus on the hearing person.
> ➤ If someone doesn't understand what you've said try saying it in a different way instead.
> ➤ Check that the person you're talking to can follow you. Be patient and take the time to communicate properly.
> ➤ Use plain language and avoid jargon and unfamiliar abbreviations.

Figure 7.1 Communicating with the deaf or hard of hearing.

speaker, typing the words phonetically, that is how they sound rather than how they are spelt. Everything that is typed appears on a computer screen. By typing in this way, the reporter can keep up with the speed of spoken English.

People who are blind or partially sighted

As with other seldom-heard groups, the methods of a research study may need to be refined to capture the diversity of strengths and needs of blind or partially sighted people. Researchers therefore need to be aware of adequately costing for additional resources and time required for recruitment and providing multimedia forms of information, such as large print, audio tape and Braille.

Most large voluntary organisations for blind people can provide visual awareness training for researchers, or provide advice and support designed to raise awareness of the needs of blind and partially sighted people. Training often covers how to effectively communicate with blind and partially sighted people – from giving directions to preparing written material – techniques for guiding visually impaired people around, and information on mobility aids, environment awareness, legislation and types of eye conditions.

People with learning disabilities

When working with people who have learning disabilities, finding ways to effectively listen is a key issue. Researchers need to think about how they will communicate with each service user, their carers and family members. The Hearing from the Seldom-Heard project which ran from April 2008 until March 2009 was funded by the Department of

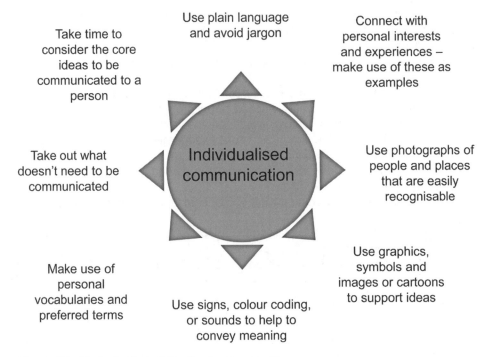

Figure 7.2   Strategies for individualised communication.

Health and undertaken by the British Institute of Learning Disabilities (BILD 2009). It aimed to look at how to overcome barriers and create listening cultures within organisations to hear from those who are seldom-heard. Six areas of good practice were identified, which are relevant to involving service users in research organisations:

- Getting to know people really well
- Better communication
- Raising awareness of the human rights of people who are seldom heard
- Improved access to advocacy
- Ensuring everyone has their own complaints buddy
- Effective complaints procedures

Other research involving people with learning disability in determining health outcomes and quality of life has used individualised communication for interviewing (Cambridge and Forrester Jones 2003). As illustrated by Figure 7.2, individualised communication involves using personal vocabularies, along with signs, graphic symbols and photographs to supplement spoken language. Collaboration with communication and speech and language therapists can also help researchers to develop a personal and flexible communication strategy for each individual service user.

Another key issue when involving people with learning disabilities is that it can be harder to explain the purpose of involvement and what it means in practical terms. Burke et al. (2003) report on the initial setting up of a participatory research project that included adults with learning disabilities, clinicians, a researcher from a primary care trust, and support workers. The authors argue that providing people with an understanding of what would be involved was important at an initial stage. In their research, people involved in undertaking a similar research project were invited to a one-day conference to talk to potential volunteers about their experiences. This helped participants to understand how they might be involved in the research.

Other researchers have argued that 'if we are concerned to include people with learning difficulties as researchers, it makes good sense to include them in the debates about the research process' (Williams and England 2005).

People with degenerative cognitive impairment

Social care research has much to offer in its use of techniques to involve people with cognitive impairment in research. For example, previous research that has involved people with dementia in research and evaluation of health services draws attention to important issues about the ethics of involvement, consent, communication and the impact of involvement (Cheston et al. 2000; Hubbard et al. 2003; Wilkinson et al. 2003). Some social care research has also argued that people who might be excluded from research studies because of difficulties in obtaining informed consent and so on may be able to participate in research if methods are tailored to their circumstances. Two examples of such methodological initiatives are Cooke's (2003) use of video among people with dementia and *Talking Mats* developed at the University of Stirling (Joseph Rowntree Foundation 2010).

A review to investigate studies that actively engage older people with dementia in research (Cowdell 2006) shows that researchers have used a range of methods to ensure that studies are ethical, meaningful and preserve the personhood of individuals. However, the skill with which this aim was achieved varied considerably from formulaic approaches to those that clearly demonstrate that the researchers have a mindset that is grounded in a powerful belief in, and application of, the concepts of genuine respect for older people with dementia. The authors draw examples of good practice from 22 studies included in the review, which have direct application to future research involving people with dementia.

People with mental health problems

People with mental health problems have traditionally been excluded from making decisions about their own welfare and the services that are provided for them (Wallcraft et al. 2009). Mental health service users can suffer stigma because of the following:

- *Public stigma* occurs when healthcare providers, employers and the general public develop and sustain negative stereotypes about people with mental illness.
- *Self-stigma* occurs when individuals with mental illness apply negative stereotypes to themselves.

• *Institutional stigma* occurs when assumptions about persons with mental health problems are translated into public policy and funding decisions that discriminate against people with mental illness.

Despite these barriers, mental health research is one of the most developed areas for service user involvement and there are several good introductory texts available in this field (see further reading in Chapter 12). The *Handbook of Service User Involvement in Mental Health Research* (Wallcraft et al. 2009) explains the influence of the mental health service user/survivor movement in the reform of mental health services, policy and the psychiatric system. The handbook also provides good practice guidance in service user involvement in mental health, including the following recommendations for laying the foundations for involvement:

• Be aware of and honest about what you expect from service user involvement.
• Carefully consider the level of involvement you aim for at each specific stage of your research project.
• Be aware of additional resources needed to take into account the time and money required to involve people fully.
• Specifically consider planning for:
  – Flexibility and periods of absence
  – Adequate support for service users: practical, emotional and research related
  – Training in relevant knowledge and skills for both service users and researchers.
• Particularly in large institutions, communicate well in advance with the Finance department and Human Resources department about your intention to involve or employ mental health service users in research – in order to facilitate the process and pre-empt any difficulties that may arise.

The research evidence for service user involvement in mental health service development and research is also well developed when compared to service user involvement in nursing and healthcare research. A review of evidence from comparative studies on the effects of involving users in the delivery and evaluation of mental health services synthesised five randomised controlled trials and seven other comparative studies (Simpson and House 2002). The findings suggest that users of mental health services can be involved as employees of such services, trainers or researchers without damaging them. In some studies, benefits were gained for clients of employees who were or who had been users of services. Interviewers who had been service users may have brought out negative opinions of services that would not otherwise have been obtained. All of the studies included in the review included details of the support provided to service users, including training and payment for involvement.

   The main issue for nursing and healthcare research is to recognise that mental health service users are a seldom-heard group, but that there is good evidence to show that they can be successfully involved as employees, trainers or researchers in the evaluation and development of services. The following case study (Box 7.2) explains how creative techniques can be a useful way of helping service users to express their views in research.

Box 7.2 Involving people with mental health problems in research

Case study

Christine Wilson, Research Fellow in Health Professional Education

I started my early research career at the Institute of Psychiatry, King's College London. In 2006 I moved to Wales and joined the Faculty of Health, Sport and Science, at the University of Glamorgan. I work within the faculty's simulation centre (http://hesas.glam.ac.uk/simulation) and have a real interest in helping patients and carers to have a voice in the research process.

Empowerment and research training

To develop a strategy for service user involvement across the Faculty I was involved in running a day-workshop at the Glamorgan Business Centre for service users, carers, healthcare educationalists and health and social care researchers. The event generated a great many ideas, including that patients and carers wanted to be more involved in 'disseminating research findings' back to their local community. We wrote an academic report about the workshop (1) and one workshop attendee, a mental health service user (JE), agreed to work with me to produce a lay report. Initially, a few hours a week were set aside to allow JE to tell his own story of using mental health services as a step towards taking an active role in writing the lay report. We used an array of creative writing and personal development techniques as a basis for the empowerment training including short stories, poems and a short video diary. Following the publication of the lay report, the empowerment and research training was offered to a larger group of mental health service users. These service users decided to form their own group – The SURE Group. Members of SURE wrote and disseminated their own short report which outlined their research aspirations and included some of their poems and short stories.

A Living Library

In early 2008 CRC-Cymru asked if I would facilitate a workshop on the benefits of providing service users with empowerment and research training at a conference for health and social care researchers. I thought the best way for researchers to understand the benefits of empowerment training would be to speak directly with the mental health service user who had received the training. The workshop was entitled '*A Living Library: Just how do researchers empower mental health service users in research?*'

The Living Library concept originated in Denmark in 2000. It offers a deliberative involvement structure that is inclusive and raises awareness of existing prejudices and unequal power relationships. It helps people to learn more about real world experience and encourages discussion and the sharing of viewpoints with others. A 'living book' may be experts in their field, have a particular passion or hobby, or have significant experiences to share. A 'reader' is anyone with an interest in gaining a greater understanding of a particular topic or theme.

With the help of The SURE Group I planned the first Living Library in Wales. We discussed the types of stories members were prepared to share and a 'book cover' was developed for each person with 'chapter titles' such as, 'Research training – what it has meant to me?' and 'Why I want to be fully involved in research'. In May 2008 at the event in Bridgend, the 'readers' were invited to loan a book for a very brief 7 min so that they could read a number of different 'books' during the workshop. In the last session we turned the tables on the researchers and asked them to become a 'living book'. Although this took them by surprise it worked very well and service users learnt from the experience too. This is what one member had to say:

> It was a unique and very exciting experience for everyone in the group. It had never been tried before so Christine said that no one would know if we made mistakes and got things wrong, as we were the only ones there that actually knew how it was

supposed to be performed! But we shouldn't have been worried, as it went perfectly. It was a very good way to meet and talk with people we wouldn't normally talk and meet with. In the workshop we learned more about what it was like to be a 'researcher' and researchers were able to learn more about us – as empowered patients. It was exciting and it helped us to break down barriers – everyone learned a lot and we enjoyed ourselves very much. (Participant in the Living Library)

Members of The SURE Group have now formed the first All Wales Service User and Carer Led Research Group and have secured funding to write their own research proposals.

Issues to be aware of:

- Service users may feel uncertain about being involved in research or unsure how they can make a contribution.
- Researchers need to understand the 'empowering' aspects of giving people with marginalised voices the opportunity to find a voice, speak up and challenge stereotypes and prejudice.

Helpful ideas:

- Creative techniques such as poetry, writing and video diaries can be a way of helping service users to gain authority over their own narrative. This in turn helps to build self-confidence and greater involvement in the research process generally.
- A Living Library is a good way to help service users to share their experiences with researchers. It can be very powerful but needs to be well organised and facilitated:
  - Help the 'living books' to define their boundaries' so that they do not attempt to talk about things that are currently emotionally painful or difficult to deal with.
  - Set up the room so there is plenty of space between tables.
  - Provide written instructions and keep people on track.
  - Allow 10–15 min for each reader to spend with each living book.
  - Invite 'readers' to handle the 'books' with care, as they are new, first editions and other people will want to read them after they have!
  - Always hold a 'debriefing session' just in case sensitive issues have been raised.

(1) Yeomans, A., Wilson, C., and Kirk, M. (2007) *Getting Involved in Research: Patient and Public Involvement*. Pontypridd, U.K.: University of Glamorgan.

Black and minority ethnic groups

Although mainstream service user participation in health care and research has increased over the last 20 years, participation of black and minority ethnic (BME) people has diminished over this period of time. Even though there is no evidence to suggest these service users do not want to participate in research, BME service users of social care (SCIE 2006) have reported feeling that

- Mainstream services are often inappropriate for them.
- Professionals make assumptions about them based on stereotypes and prejudice.
- There are language barriers.
- Religious and cultural identity is rarely responded to by mainstream service providers.

BME groups can also suffer from what is sometimes referred to as double or triple discrimination (Chahal and Uklah 2004). For example, families from BME communities who are caring for someone with a physical or learning disability face the same difficulties as other people but these problems are compounded by additional factors. These factors might include racism, health inequalities and language barriers, stereotypical views of black people, stigma and cultural ignorance (Sainsbury Centre for Mental Health 2004).

As well as having benefits for research processes and outcomes, involvement of BME groups in health and social care research can help to:

- Overcome prejudice
- Support integration
- Improve cohesion of communities in society (SCIE 2006)

Researchers may need to make specific adjustments to the way they work to ensure that the needs of BME groups and newly arrived communities are considered. For example, the majority of research with BME communities shows that language is a barrier and that research teams need to translate written materials or use translators to support involvement. However, there is an argument that translation should not be used as a substitute for learning local languages (SCIE 2006). While many research organisations have produced information in community languages, there has sometimes been little uptake from the communities they are aimed at. There are also many decisions to be made at the point of translation, including what to translate, which languages to choose and how to ensure the quality of translation. Despite these issues, access to language translation services is beneficial for any research organisation.

Relatively little attention has been paid to involving BME groups in research about culturally sensitive subjects. One notable exception is research on the enablement of ethnic minority groups to participate in research about cervical screening (Chiu 2004). This work shows that issues of stigma and confidentiality can be considerable barriers to involving BME groups in health research.

Key principles for practice

- Researchers should take time to consider the multiple barriers and circumstances that seldom-heard groups face including lack of awareness, communication barriers and access issues.
- Researchers should pay careful attention to individual needs and access to working environments to ensure that people with physical disabilities can be involved.
- Researchers should consider the communication preferences of the deaf and people who are hard of hearing, for example using lip-reading, sign language, and large screen projection of speech-to-text.
- In order to successfully involve people who are blind or partially sighted, researchers need to adequately cost for additional resources and time required for recruitment, providing multimedia forms of information, and for researcher visual awareness training.
- Researchers who plan to work with people who have learning disabilities need to find ways to effectively communicate with each service user, their carers and family members.

This could involve using personal vocabularies, along with signs, graphic symbols and photographs to supplement spoken language.
- Researchers who intend to involve people with cognitive impairment in research should pay particular attention to the ethics of involvement, consent, communication and the impact of involvement.
- Researchers should be aware that mental health service users are a seldom-heard group but that they can be successfully involved as employees, trainers or researchers in the evaluation and development of services.
- Researchers should seek to inform themselves about the types of issues that black and minority ethnic groups may suffer, including racism, health inequalities and language barriers.

References

British Institute of Learning Disability (BILD) (2009) *Hearing from the Seldom Heard*. Kidderminster: British Institute of Learning Disability.

Burke, A., McMillan, J., Cummins, L., Thompson, A., Forsyth, W., McLellan, J. et al. (2003) Setting up participatory research: A discussion of the initial stages. *British Journal of Learning Disabilities*, 31 (2): 65–9.

Cambridge, P. and Forrester-Jones, R. (2003) Using individualised communication for interviewing people with intellectual disability: a case study of user-centred research. *Journal of Intellectual & Developmental Disability*, 28 (1): 5–23.

Chahal, K. and Ullah, A. (2004) *Experiencing Ethnicity: Discrimination and Service Provision*. York: Joseph Rowntree Foundation.

Cheston, R., Bender, M., and Byatt, S. (2000) Involving people who have dementia in the evaluation of services, a review. *Journal of Mental Health*, 9 (5): 471–9.

Chiu, L. (2004) Minority ethnic women and cervical screening: a matter of action or research? *Primary Health Care Research & Development*, 5(2): 104–16.

Cooke, A. (2003) Using video to include the experiences of older people with dementia in research. *Research Policy & Planning*, 21 (2): 23–32.

Cowdell, F. (2006) Preserving personhood in dementia research: a literature review. *International Journal of Older People Nursing*, 1 (2): 85–94.

Hubbard, G., Down, M., and Tester, S. (2003) Including older people with dementia in research: challenges and strategies. *Aging & Mental Health*, 7: 351–62.

Joseph Rowntree Foundation (2010) *Talking Mats Help Involve People with Dementia and Their Carers in Decision-Making*. York: Joseph Rowntree Foundation.

Sainsbury Centre for Mental Health (2004) *Breaking the Circles of Fear: A Review of the Relationship between Mental Health Services and African and Caribbean Communities*. London: Sainsbury Centre for Mental Health.

Simpson, E. and House, A. (2002) Involving users in the delivery and evaluation of mental health services: systematic review. *British Medical Journal*, 325: 1265.

Social Care Institute for Excellence (SCIE) (2006) *Doing It for Themselves: Participation and Black and Minority Ethnic Service Users*. London: Social Care Institute for Excellence.

Social Care Institute for Excellence (SCIE) (2008) *Seldom Heard: Developing Inclusive Participation in Social Care*. London: Social Care Institute for Excellence.

Steel, R. (2005) Actively involving marginalized and vulnerable people in research. In: Lowes, L. and Hulatt, I. (eds) *Involving Service Users in Health and Social Care Research*. London: Routledge.

Wallcraft, J., Schrank, B., and Amering, M. (2009) *Handbook of Service User Involvement in Mental Health Research*. World Psychiatric Association. West Sussex: Wiley-Blackwell.

Wilkinson, H., Bowes, A., and Rodrigues, A. (2003) Innovative methodologies – can we learn from including people with dementia from South Asian communities. *Research Policy & Planning* 21 (2): 43–54.

Williams, V. and England, M. (2005) Supporting people with learning difficulties to do their own research. In: Lowes, L. and Hulatt, I. (eds) *Involving Service Users in Health and Social Care Research*. London: Routledge.

Chapter 8

Service user-led research

> **Key summary points**
>
> - *Personal health research*: Personal health research could be described as individual service users, sometimes with the help of their family members or carers, undertaking their own research to better understand an illness or the options for treatment or care. For service users and their relatives learning about their health status can be an essential step towards achieving improved health, understanding or acceptance of a health condition.
> - *Volunteer networks*: Volunteers contribute in many different roles to the delivery of health and social care services, including supporting research activity. As members of volunteer networks, service users may undertake their own research or use research findings to lobby for change and bring about action.
> - *Service user-led organisations*: Many service users organise themselves into self-help, support or interest groups. They may investigate health issues and can be powerful advocates for research into particular health conditions or health services.
> - *Charities and not-for-profit organisations*: Charitable organisations may directly commission and fund research from charitable donations. Many produce accessible information about research findings and provide a point of access for service users to information about ongoing research studies.
> - *Experienced service user representatives*: Service users can become experienced service user representatives who may be involved in a range of public and professional domains. There are many advantages to involving experienced service user representatives in research, for example they may be aware of a range of health issues or knowledgeable about local health service provision and have an understanding of the relative importance of health issues to different groups of service users.
> - *Academic service user researchers*: In recent years some academic departments, particularly in mental health and social care research, have appointed service users as members of staff. Academic service user researchers bring many of the advantages associated with service user involvement, as well as advantages associated with continuity of experience and normalising service user involvement.

Handbook of Service User Involvement in Nursing and Healthcare Research, First Edition.
Elizabeth Morrow, Annette Boaz, Sally Brearley and Fiona Ross.
© 2012 Elizabeth Morrow, Annette Boaz, Sally Brearley and Fiona Ross.
Published 2012 by Blackwell Publishing Ltd.

Personal health research

Personal health research could be described as individual service users, sometimes with the help of their family members or carers, undertaking their own research to better understand an illness or the options for treatment or care. It is an aspect of nursing and healthcare research that often goes unrecognised, largely because it is unfunded, may not use established research methods, or be written in a scholarly fashion. Yet, for service users and their relatives learning about their health status can be an essential step towards achieving improved health, understanding or acceptance of a health condition. There are similarities between personal health research and emancipatory approaches to research (see Chapter 3, 'Building in opportunities for involvement' section). In both, service users aim to gain a better insight into their own situation in order to improve things for themselves. In the UK, the notion of 'survivor research' has also become popular, particularly in mental health research, to mean people are survivors of their own distress or of the negative aspects of service use they may have experienced (Sweeney et al. 2009).

As the following case study (Box 8.1) illustrates, service users can become experts in their own right, to the extent that they are able to offer valuable insights to healthcare professionals.

In the context of moves towards increased personal responsibility and choice over health care in many countries, definitions of personal health research need to be debated and shared more widely. In mental health research, Strategies for Living (Faulkner 2000) was a qualitative study involving interviews with 71 mental health service users. Designed and executed by service users, the research explored people's strategies for living and coping with mental distress. The predominant theme to emerge concerned the importance of relationships with others, especially family and friends, and people encountered at day centres and self-help groups. Peer support, the support of others in similar circumstances and the value of self-help received warm and grateful praise. This suggests that practitioners should pay more attention to the role of self-help and peer support in overcoming stigma and discrimination. Mental health professionals should facilitate self-management, rather than prioritising interventions aimed at symptom eradication. Ideas such as the Expert Patients Programme (EPP) in the UK can help to equip service users with the skills to understand their own health better. EPP is a self-management programme for people who are living with a long-term health condition such as arthritis, asthma and diabetes. The basis of the programme is a training course that teaches people how to manage their conditions by using problem-solving, decision-making, making the best use of resources, developing effective partnerships with healthcare providers and taking appropriate action. Linking service users with programmes like these and providing support for personal health research are likely to become stronger features of nursing and healthcare practice in the future.

Volunteer networks

Within many health systems internationally volunteers make a huge contribution to service delivery. It is increasingly recognised that volunteers add substantial value to

Box 8.1   Patients and families who do their own research

Case study

The Sunderland Family

I'm Shirley and I work for the adult careers service in the North East. My sister Joanne works for Northumberland Care Trust. We lost our lovely father to Mesothelioma (Meso) in March 2009. This cancer is caused by exposure to asbestos. It is killing more people than ever before and numbers are expected to peak in 2017.

Issue/Scenario:

My dad, Ken Sunderland, was diagnosed with Mesothelioma in 2006. He was exposed to asbestos in the 1960s and 1970s when he tested and commissioned heating and ventilation systems on ships. At the outset, the only option offered to him was chemotherapy. He was fortunate to be living in an area where Alimta (the chemo drug) was available, but we were all concerned about the lack of other options available, especially Dad, one of those people who wanted to understand and know as much about his disease as possible.

So Dad, Jo and I trawled the internet for anything and everything to do with Meso. We found out about trials and alternative treatments (including some pretty strange ones) going on across the globe – and many that were closer to home – such as Meso conferences, clinical trials, local groups and charities. It was a full-time job keeping on top of what was being written about Meso treatments and research. We were in touch (by email and phone) with leading Meso clinicians and surgeons in the UK, Australia, America and Germany about standard and more pioneering treatments. There was no such information coming from Dad's hospital, and there was no central signposting resource. The Alimta kept Dad's Meso in check for a while, but the side effects of the drugs were sometimes very hard for him to bear. Through Jo's research, we found a trial in Germany involving a process called chemo-embolisation whereby chemotherapy is administered directly into the tumour via the arterial system. It was working well for a Meso sufferer he befriended from Plymouth. In late 2008, Dad was provided with his lung scans and he sent them to Germany. Together, our parents made the trip to Frankfurt (consultation, scans, results, treatment and care – all excellent and done in just 3 days): funded himself at a cost of £3,000. Dad wanted to try, and would never have had the choice if we had not done the research ourselves. Scans showed that the tumour had reduced in size after the Germany trip, but tragically for Dad it was too little, too late. He passed away at home in March 2009 with all of us by his side.

Dad wrote a diary. He wanted to share some messages with medical professionals. Here they are:

- Patients need a single point of contact to find out all they need to know about this disease and the options open to them (perhaps the proposed National Centre for Asbestos-Related Disease could act as this point, a hub, for all information dissemination – for what is happening in the UK and also across the rest of the world). This point of contact needs to be able to cater for a wide spectrum of patients with different attitudes, views and information needs.
- Take a holistic approach when dealing with patients and avoid focusing solely on your area of expertise.
- Think about how you speak to patients, what you say and how you say it; how would you want to be spoken to?
- Be guided in your communications by the level of knowledge that the patient has, needs and actually wants. If they want lots of information, a 10 min consultation slot is not appropriate.
- Show willingness to embrace and explore new technologies and developments and not dismiss them out of hand.

- Acknowledge that some patients know just as much as oncologists about their own cancer and potential treatments. View consultations as a two-way learning process.
- Deliver care that takes into account the individual and diverse needs of each patient.

If you'd like to read Dad's full account you can find it at: http://www.mickknightonmesorf.org/your-stories/ken-sunderlands-diary/

publically funded health services. In countries with a public health system there can be hundreds of different roles open to volunteers, from assisting with administration and meeting and greeting to holding patients' hands during eye operations, or simply taking the time to sit and chat to patients who may not have any family or friends to visit. Healthcare professionals may undertake voluntary work as part of their training or practice development.

As members of volunteer networks, service users and carers often play a role in promoting and undertaking nursing and healthcare research, for example by helping to recruit patients to research studies or administering patient experience questionnaires. However, in these examples overall control of the research is maintained by professional groups who design the research and determine which questions service users will be asked.

Voluntary sector organisations are increasingly playing an important role in health care, both as providers of services, and as advocates and campaigners on behalf of those in need of better care. For example in England, National Voices is the umbrella organisation established by and for the voluntary sector, and in Scotland Voluntary Health Scotland is the national intermediary body for voluntary health organisations. Organisations such as these bring together all national voluntary organisations representing users of health and social care to give them a stronger voice in policy-making and other professional arenas. The collective efforts of volunteers working through such organisations, contributes to healthcare research by influencing health and social care policy and planning as well as having a direct influence on healthcare professionals and researchers.

As members of volunteer networks service users may undertake their own research or use research findings to lobby for change and bring about action. Often organisations will survey their members to elicit healthcare issues, to find out about problems they are facing, or to generate suggestions for change. In the UK, the Alzheimer's Society is a pioneer in public involvement in dementia research. The society Research Network is a team of over 180 carers, former carers and people with dementia. Research Network volunteers play an integral role in the research programme by setting research priorities, assessing and commenting on grant applications, monitoring ongoing projects funded by Alzheimer's Society and telling other people about the results of research.

Service user-led organisations

Many service users organise themselves into self-help, support or interest groups. A service user-led organisation is run and controlled by people who use health and/or social care services, including people with physical or learning disabilities, mental health service users, older people and their families and carers. Service user-led organisations provide advocacy, peer support, and information and advice on issues such as personal budgets, personal payments for social care, self-assessment, support planning and employing personal assistants. They also work with statutory and other agencies to develop strategies for improving services. They may investigate health issues and can be powerful advocates for research into particular health conditions, service provision, or strategies for living with illness (Nicholls 2001). Carers may also be involved in, or take responsibility for, determining the direction of research that service user-led organisations undertake.

Service user-led organisations have highlighted two activities as central to making service user involvement work (Branfield and Beresford 2006). These are: people being able to get together to work collectively for change and mutual support, and the importance of making known their own experience, views and ideas. This is because service user organisations and individual service users are often isolated. The closed culture of health and social care services and their own inadequate resources often restrict service users' capacity to develop and share their knowledge. Service user-led groups may experience difficulties attracting long-term funding and managing the resources they do have because of a lack of financial management and business development skills.

As discussed in Chapter 1, user-led and user-controlled research concerns research processes as much as research outcomes. Service user-led organisations can enable service users to take part in research education or training, or to carry out research, while gaining skills and confidence in the process (Faulkner and Thomas 2002). Some service user-led organisations that provide advice and support about service user involvement in research include the following:

- *Shaping Our Lives National User Network* is an independent user-controlled organisation since 2002. The network aims to improve the quality of services and support people receive particularly in social care. The website supports service user organisations, service users and others who are interested in developing service user involvement at local and national levels and to allow links to develop between user-controlled groups. It provides links to a range of resources and publications including guidelines and practical support for involving users.
- *HelpYourselves.org.uk* aims to give support to young people wishing to be involved and to practitioners wishing to involve young people. It provides skills for young people to take up opportunities to speak out on issues that affect them. The website includes tools to help young people to develop local projects. The resources in their extensive list are aimed at involving young people but include good practice guides and a wide range of resources that can be adapted for use with most groups. The website also includes practical toolkits and guides.

In mental health research service user organisations have made a real difference using a collective voice and research findings to bring about changes in service provision. User-Focused Monitoring (UFM) was first developed and pioneered by the Sainsbury Centre for Mental Health in 1997 with a pilot user-run project in the London Borough of Kensington & Chelsea and Westminster (Rose 2001). Mental health service users with severe and enduring mental health problems created, developed, carried out and analysed the research. Some 61 user interviewers were trained and they interviewed over 500 service users living both in the community, and in hospital on seven sites situated in urban, rural and seaside areas of England. The fact that the questions were developed and asked by user interviewers is important and affected the interviewee's responses as interviewees reported they had 'been through the system' and understood their own situation. The research was important because it showed that people with mental health problems are perfectly capable of judging the services they receive.

The following case study (Box 8.2) illustrates how working in collaboration with members of support groups and networks can help to sustain service user efforts.

Charities and not-for-profit organisations

Charities and not-for-profit organisations can be involved in, or lead, research related to nursing or health care. They may directly commission and fund research from charitable donations, including reviewing proposals for research or providing personal awards to nurse researchers. Not-for-profit organisations, which can include charities, do not distribute their surplus funds to owners or shareholders, but instead use them to help pursue their goals, which may include research. In most countries, not-for-profit organisations are exempt from income and property taxation. Many health charities and not-for-profit organisations produce accessible information about research findings and may also provide a point of access for service users to information about ongoing research studies. The UK charity sector is distinct internationally in terms of its scale and impact. Approximately one third of all public expenditure on medical and health research in the UK comes from the medical research charities. Sources of further information include the following:

- *The Association of Medical Research Charities* (AMRC) is a membership organisation of the leading medical and health research charities in the UK. AMRC aims to support the sector's effectiveness and advance medical research by developing best practice, providing information and guidance, improving public dialogue about research and science, and influencing government. Formally established in 1987, AMRC has 125 member charities that contribute over £1 billion annually to medical research aimed at tackling diseases such as heart disease, cancer and diabetes, as well as rarer conditions like cystic fibrosis and motor neurone disease.
- *The UK Charities Directory* is a support service to charity and non-profit-making organisations. The Charities Directory online (www.charitydirectory.com) includes free list of charities, non-profit-making organisations, a message board and charity newsletter.
- *User involvement in research – a route map* is designed for staff who work in health research charities and other organisations that commission or fund research who wish to involve service users in their work. It provides advice on where to start as well as lessons from organisations that have already involved service users. There are examples of forms, policies and strategies that you can download and adapt for your own use (www.twocanassociates.co.uk).

Box 8.2   Moving forward and sustaining collective service user efforts

Case study

Nazira Visram

I am an experienced patient representative with a wide range of involvements including being a Macmillan Trainer, contributing to experiential learning and self-management programmes for cancer care. Some of my involvement includes chairing a local support group, facilitating a support group on south London, chairing the breast cancer care service user research partnership group, patient representative on the connected expert advisory group, involvement in the survivorship agenda in the consequences of treatments work stream. My involvement varies considerably as it can be local, national and international. I speak at conferences from a service user perspective and I have had opportunities to deliver master classes on service user involvement.

Issue: 'Finding windows of opportunity'

In my experience as a service user representative, engaging at all different levels is essential. At the grass-root level needs are constantly changing and it is vital to ensure these needs are represented at national level where decisions are made. In my experience over the last few years, cancer services have gone from strength to strength and this has been due to the dedication of the people who work in that setting together with the opportunity given to patients and carers to make recommendations about the changing needs. When the cancer plan was introduced in 2000 'partnership working' was a terminology – it is now becoming a reality. It isn't always a smooth run and often good ideas do go into limbo purely due to inappropriate timing. This can cause frustration and it can be difficult to keep the momentum going. Let me explain this through an example. About 4 months after my clinical treatment, I attended a talk on Lymphoedema which flagged up concerns for me. Through referral it was confirmed that I had early stages of Lymphoedema in my left arm. This is a condition that can come about following cancer investigation procedures or due to radiotherapy/surgery – there are many factors involved. This was an outcome of cancer. At first sight it does not seem too much of an issue compared to cancer diagnosis though patients with the condition will confirm that it robs individuals of quality of life. Being able to live a life having survived cancer is equally important.

Anyway I was given relevant information, hosiery and told that my condition would be reviewed in a month's time. Upon returning back I discovered that the Lymphoedema nurse had moved to another job and that I would be seen in the interim by my CNS. Although supportive, she was limited in what she could offer as it was not her area of expertise. It took a fair time before another therapist took up that role highlighting yet another concern. Having one therapist was inadequate due to the level of physical care involved, resulting in inequality and restricted service. On occasions when she was on annual leave or sick, things came to a standstill. Patients felt abandoned due to lack of continuity. It led to frustration all round.

Upon reflection it was apparent that the service needed two therapists in order to run effectively. Starting up a Lymphoedema support group followed, which identified the number of people requiring this service. Joint input in putting together a case led to a successful outcome. We now have an effective service; however, it is also vital to remember that reaching our goal took not months but years. At the time when we identified a need, the focus was on other aspects of cancer care and this was when things went into limbo – by the time we were successful, the focus was turning onto the cancer reform strategy and survivorship. We now have to work towards sustaining this service by collecting research evidence to show the benefits of the service in the long run.

I have learnt over the years that we have to make best use of small windows of opportunity that come about. It's about getting all relevant information together and using the opportunity when it arises.

Key issues to be aware of:

- Service user involvement requires a lot of energy, passion, enthusiasm, time and determination.
- Service users can make a difference using a collective voice on various issues through support groups and cancer networks.
- Service users may have strong views about a particular health issue or a service and these are often basic changes that don't necessarily require extensive funding.
- A lot of changes are politically driven, bringing with it confusion for both service users and professionals.
- Including service users at the planning stage of a service can in fact be cost-effective and can result in genuine partnership.
- It is essential to keep focus on the existing needs as they continue to exist alongside the new ones that get identified.

Helpful ideas:

- Partnership working brings together relevant skills and qualities.
- Organisations such as Macmillan Cancer Support offer support through workshops in working together effectively.
- It is essential to be aware of new policy initiatives and use them to drive work forward.

Experienced service user representatives

Service users can become experienced service user representatives who may be involved in a range of public and professional domains. For example, service users may also be community representatives, members of regional councils, leaders of voluntary organisations, members of parent teacher associations, members of carer organisations, leaders within a religious community, non-executive board members for a local healthcare provider, or users of multiple health and social care services. It is not unusual for experienced service users to hold multiple roles at any one time which can mean they are well connected to different community groups and provide a bridging role into different professional arenas. They may have developed a good understanding of the different ways of working and the way in which decisions are made in different social arenas.

There are many advantages to involving experienced service user representatives in research, for example they may:

- Be aware of a range of health issues or knowledgeable about local health service provision;
- Have an understanding of the relative importance of health issues to different groups of service users;
- Have the confidence and experience to communicate research issues to professionals and members of the public;
- Be recognised as a community/patient representative;
- Be able to access different groups of the public, for example to support the recruitment of participants or the dissemination of research to service users;
- Understand how different service users or groups of the community are likely to relate to one another, and to healthcare professionals;

• Have research skills and experience, including experience of applying for research funding and publishing research findings.

We should not forget that, like any other people, professional researchers and healthcare professionals can become service users. In circumstances where researchers become ill or need to make use of health services, their prior research experience can be beneficial for identifying issues that research could potentially address. However, becoming ill, or being admitted as an inpatient, can be a daunting experience for anyone and professionals may wish to keep their own experiences personal and private. They may also feel it is not appropriate to mix their professional and personal lives as a researcher and a service user.

Academic service user researchers

In recent years some academic departments, particularly in mental health and social care research, have appointed service users as members of staff. Employing service users on fixed-term or permanent posts has the advantage of building experience and knowledge within a department. It can also help individual service users to build a research career. In Australia 'academic consumer researchers' have been shown to increase the relevance of mental health research to service users, to bridge the gap between the academic and service user communities and to contribute to the process of destigmatising mental disorders (Griffiths et al. 2003).

Good practice guidance has been devised for employing service users in mental health research, which includes advice on researcher preparation, hiring service users, salary payments, training, supervision, support, and team building, as well as creating opportunities for involvement at all stages and attaining additional resources to support these activities (Delman and Lincoln 2009). In the following case study (Box 8.3) a user-researcher explains their role within a university department in England and provides some helpful ideas about tackling stigma and discrimination towards mental health service users.

To date, in many countries there has been little recognition of the particular contributions that service users with formal academic qualifications and research experience can offer. Academic service user researchers bring many of the advantages associated with service user involvement, as well as further benefits associated with continuity of experience, for example forming close working relationships with members of a research team. Involving service users as part of the academic culture also helps to normalise service user involvement in research (Delman and Lincoln 2009). Figure 8.1 illustrates these and some other potential advantages.

An example of an academic unit that has led the way in employing service users is the Service User Research Enterprise (SURE) based at the Institute of Psychiatry at King's College London. SURE was launched in 2001 and it is now one of the largest units within universities in Europe to employ people who have both research skills and first-hand experience of mental health services and treatments. SURE undertakes research that tests the effectiveness of services and treatments from the perspective of people with mental health problems and their carers. It aims to involve service users in a collaborative way in the whole research process, from design to data collection, through to data analysis and

Box 8.3   Service user involvement from a user-researcher's perspective

Case study

Rory Byrne

I'm a user-researcher based at the University of Manchester, working in Psychology. I'm involved in a number of large-scale research projects at the moment including two major research trials of cognitive therapy for psychosis. My role includes conducting user-led interviews with participants in those trials to assess their experiences before and after involvement. Another research project I'm developing will be aimed at assessing service users' preferences and priorities for treatment of psychosis. Along with those aspects of my role, I've also given quite a few presentations at meetings and conferences, both describing my own experience and presenting other research.

Personal experience leading to professional understanding

I have experience of becoming 'at risk' of psychosis, and of receiving cognitive therapy (rather than anti-psychotic medication) to prevent full onset, which was successful. My experience of using services, therefore, has been far less difficult than for many other people. In particular, I was very fortunate to have been involved with mental health professionals who were primarily focused on *normalising* my psychological problems and promoting my *recovery*. In my personal and professional experience, the issue of stigma and discrimination associated with psychosis is one of the greatest difficulties people face when becoming unwell, and even after they've become involved with services. In fact, there's strong evidence to show that many mental health professionals can stigmatise service users as much, or more, than members of the general population, especially through narrow adherence to the 'medical model' of psychosis. With this in mind, I think it's extremely important that the focus should always be on a normalising, recovery-focused paradigm, rather than the traditional pathologising, illness model of psychosis or schizophrenia.

Key issues to be aware of:

- A significant barrier in the way of service user involvement in research is the stigma and discrimination still so widely associated with mental health problems and with psychosis and schizophrenia in particular. Unfortunately there is strong evidence to suggest that mental health professionals may be among those most likely to stigmatise service users, and this may negatively affect service user involvement in research.
- 'Normalising' mental health problems can be an effective intervention in itself. Information and interpersonal treatment that help service users involved in nursing or healthcare research to see their psychological problems as fundamentally normal should be offered more routinely.

Helpful ideas:

- Healthcare professionals and researchers should undertake anti-stigma education and training to understand how to tackle stigma and discrimination.
- An effective way to reduce stigma is through 'contact interventions'; positive experiences of one-to-one contact with members of a stigmatised group that can dispel the unfounded concerns that underlie prejudice, and highlight the positive value of users' personal involvement with other mental health service stakeholders.
- Another solution to stigma is to increase the number of service users included as members of clinical teams, research teams, and mental health service provision in general.

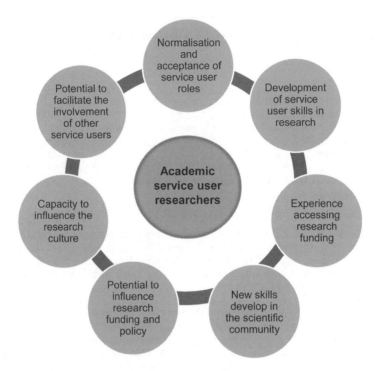

Figure 8.1   Potential advantages of employing academic service user researchers.

dissemination of results (Rose 2003). The unit has two co-directors, a service user researcher and a clinical academic, which adds balance to the management structure.

In mental health research, good practice guidance has been developed for employment of service user researchers (Wallcraft et al. 2009):

- Develop a clear and realistic job description, highlighting the essential job functions and minimal qualifications necessary.
- Distribute the job notice widely; include user groups and diverse community groups.
- Interview job applicants in teams including at least one service user.
- Be clear and realistic about the amount of control over the research project that the person to be employed will have.
- Communicate in clear language, and be aware that people with different backgrounds may understand things differently.
- Provide for a possibility for regular open discussion, formal and personal support, and for supervision.
- Make clear arrangements about who to talk to and where to turn in case of personal problems. This should be separate from the workplace.
- Discuss openly the possibility of the service user researcher becoming ill or unable to work and make clear arrangements in case of this happening.
- Provide for sufficient training opportunities.
- Provide for opportunities to meet up with other service user researchers and share common experiences.

Key principles for practice

- Researchers and healthcare professionals can learn from service users who undertake personal health research about their illness or the options for treatment or care.
- Researchers should consider working with volunteer networks to undertake research or to join efforts to lobby for change and bring about action.
- Researchers should be aware that service user-led organisations may investigate health issues and can be powerful advocates for research into particular health conditions or services.
- Researchers should be aware that charitable organisations may directly commission and fund research and can be an accessible source of information about research for service users.
- There are advantages to working with experienced service users, particularly to find ways to engage with different groups of service users.
- It is becoming more common for academic departments to employ service users. This helps to gain continuity of experience and normalise service user involvement.

References

Branfield F. and Beresford P. (2006) *Making User Involvement Work: Supporting Service User Networking and Knowledge*. York: Joseph Rowntree Foundation.

Delman, J. and Lincoln, A. (2009) Service users as paid researchers. In: Wallcraft, J., Schrank, B., and Amering, M. (eds) *Handbook of Service User Involvement in Mental Health Research*. Chichester: Wiley-Blackwell.

Faulkner, A. (2000) *Strategies for Living: A Report of User-Led Research into People's Strategies for Living with Mental Distress*. London: Mental Health Foundation.

Faulkner, A. and Thomas, P. (2002) User-led research and evidence based medicine. *The British Journal of Psychiatry*, 180: 1–3.

Griffiths, K., Jorm, A., and Christensen, H. (2003) Academic consumer researchers: a bridge between consumers and researchers. *Australian & New Zealand Journal of Psychiatry*, 38 (4): 191–6.

Nicholls, V. (2001) *Doing Research Ourselves*. London: Mental Health Foundation.

Rose, D. (2001) *Users' Voices: The Perspective of Mental Health Service Users on Community and Hospital Care*. London: Sainsbury Centre for Mental Health.

Rose, D. (2003) Collaborative research between users and professionals: peaks and pitfalls. *Psychology Bulletin*, 27: 404–6.

Sweeney, A., Beresford, P., Faulkner, A., Nettle, M., and Rose, D. (eds) (2009) *This Is Survivor Research*. Ross-on-Wye: PPCS Books.

Wallcraft, J., Schrank, B., and Amering, M. (2009) *Handbook of Service User Involvement in Mental Health Research*. World Psychiatric Association. West Sussex: Wiley-Blackwell.

Part III

Evaluating

Chapter 9

Quality

Key summary points

- *Indicators of successful involvement*: Research teams can indicate successful involvement by assuring that: the roles of service users in the research were documented; records of funding and reimbursement are kept; the contribution of service users' skills, knowledge and experience are included in research reports and papers; service users' and researchers' training needs and training are recorded; service users' advice about recruitment and participant information were sought and noted; the involvement of service users in the research reports and publications was acknowledged; research findings were disseminated to service users and relevant service user groups in appropriate formats and easily understandable language.
- *Documenting service user involvement work*: As part of recording research processes, researchers may need to demonstrate active and direct participation of service users in the commissioning, design, undertaking or evaluation of research. This can be achieved by keeping an activities log about what happens through the research and reporting on involvement at the end of a study or programme.
- *Using reflective techniques*: In any research study, service users and researchers can make use of a range of reflective techniques to examine issues about the quality of involvement processes. Some examples are reflective diaries, feedback and evaluation forms and reflective interviewing.
- *Reflexivity and service user involvement*: Reflexivity means using structured methods to pay attention to the personal, interpersonal, contextual, political and ethical factors which influence research. Reflexivity can help to identify the strengths and limitations of what has been done. It can make decisions behind the research more explicit and improve the transparency of research processes.
- *Quality experiences of involvement*: Research teams can work towards quality experiences of involvement by understanding the perspectives of those that are involved in the research, which could include both service users and researchers. Three areas of personal experience – ability, potential and sense of being – can be used as prompts to encourage reflection and learning about service user involvement.
- *Quality environments for involvement*: Quality involvement goes beyond the actions of individual service users or researchers to include research relationships, ways of doing

---

Handbook of Service User Involvement in Nursing and Healthcare Research, First Edition.
Elizabeth Morrow, Annette Boaz, Sally Brearley and Fiona Ross.
© 2012 Elizabeth Morrow, Annette Boaz, Sally Brearley and Fiona Ross.
Published 2012 by Blackwell Publishing Ltd.

research, and research structures. By considering these themes and drawing attention to quality at an organisational and research systems level, research teams may be more able to build more supportive research environments and to challenge any barriers to involvement. It could help organisations to tackle issues such as balancing competing pressures and priorities.

Indicators of successful involvement

In this chapter we look at issues regarding the quality of service user involvement in research. We have chosen to use the term quality because it encompasses a broad range of ideas about good practice, meaningful involvement and successful involvement. We aim to look at some of these different perspectives and to offer some tools and techniques for monitoring and promoting the quality of service user involvement in nursing and health-care research.

Service users who are considering being involved in research are likely to make their own minds up about whether the experience is positive and worthwhile. Service users may ask:

- What sort of things will I be asked to do?
- What type of time commitment will it take?
- Will things be explained to me?
- Can I choose how to be involved?
- Will I meet people that are interesting and friendly?
- Will I be treated with respect and dignity?
- Will my views and opinions count?
- Will I have to travel far?
- Will I be reimbursed or paid?
- Will I be trained?
- Will I get feedback about my involvement?
- Will things change as a result of my involvement?

In the UK, a consensus study amongst researchers and service users shows that there are certain things that research teams can do to ensure successful involvement in health research (Telford et al. 2004). Nine good practice principles have been identified with associated indicators; these are summarised in the following table as ten action points for research teams in nursing and healthcare research contexts (Box 9.1).

In social care, a study of service user involvement in five different research studies identified common factors that ensure success (Blackburn et al. 2010). These were:

- Building relationships – working in partnership with service users, showing you respect and value their expertise, showing that you are listening and making changes in response to their input.

Box 9.1 Ten action points for successful service user involvement

1. Apply for funding to involve service users
2. Reimburse travel costs and expenses (e.g. carer costs)
3. Document service user knowledge and skills in publications
4. Agree on service user's training needs and provide training
5. Provide personal and technical support to service users
6. Ensure researcher training needs are met
7. Seek service user's advice on how to recruit participants
8. Seek service user's advice on how to keep participants informed about the progress of the research
9. Provide details in research reports of how service users were involved in the research and acknowledge their contributions
10. Distribute research findings to service users who are involved and to relevant service user groups in appropriate formats and easily understandable language

---

- Going the extra mile – making an extra effort to ensure service users can be involved in a way that meets their needs, for example holding meetings outside of office hours, printing out documents for people.
- Honesty – being clear that research takes a long time and does not necessarily lead to change as well as being open and transparent about how you are working.
- Being sensitive and aware – some topics are going to be very sensitive and emotional. You need to manage this and support people appropriately at the same time as being clear about boundaries.
- Clarity about roles – taking time at the start of a project to explain what you need from the people you involve and how they can help you.
- Being mindful of the practical issues and minimising the costs for service users – the 'little things' really matter and can determine whether an individual can get involved.
- Investing a lot of time – especially when planning involvement and supporting people during the project.

Good practice guidance has been developed for service user involvement in mental health research and includes advice on: laying the foundations, capacity building, identifying research priorities, undertaking research with service users, payment and budgeting (Schrank and Wallcraft 2009).

Documenting service user involvement work

As a starting point for monitoring and promoting quality, research teams should aim to document service user involvement in the commissioning, design, undertaking or evaluation of research. There are several reasons for doing this, including:

- Reporting back to research funders about how resources for the involvement of service users have been used.
- Providing those service users who have been involved with feedback about their involvement and how it has contributed to the research.

- Explaining in a final report what type of involvement has been achieved and how processes of involvement have developed over the research.
- Undertaking an analysis of the impact of involvement of service users in the research.
- Supporting researcher professional development and learning about research practices.

It is useful to maintain a continuous record of service user involvement, for example by keeping an activities log about what happens through the research. Figure 9.1 provides an outline of some of the types of information that could be useful to record either at regular intervals (such as once a week or month) or at key points in the course of the research (such as at the end of phases or stages of the work). It may be more fitting to record different types of information about different aspects of a research study or types of involvement activities depending on the research context.

Some other issues to think about in relation to documenting service user involvement activities are:

- What information about service user involvement is it essential to collect and what is less important?
- How will the information be used, for example, to inform the research or the work of the research team?
- What time and resources are available for collating and analysing information that is collected?
- How will service users be involved in documenting their involvement in the research?
- Is it necessary to build extra time into the project time frame and apply for additional funding for this aspect of the work?

Date/ project timescale	Description of involvement achieved	Level of involvement	Persons involved	Impact on the research	Other outcomes
e.g. Recruit service user group for research project (Month 1)	Link with local community groups Promote study and involvement	Consultation	Lead researcher with support from project advisory group	Effect on membership and agenda of meetings recorded	Links made to other service user groups not previously identified
e.g. Meet training and support needs of service users involved (Month 2)	Understand and address training and support needs of service users Ask service users about their needs Seek guidance and support	Collaboration	Lead researcher with service users	Training preferences and uptake recorded	Involvement of external support groups, facilitation, and additional project team support
e.g. Feedback to service users' organisations (Month 9)	Service users involved disseminate findings to their organisations Communication of main achievements by service user's preferred method	User-led	Lead researcher with chair of service user group	Newsletters and feedback to service user organisations recorded	Publications for lay audiences extended dissemination of findings

Figure 9.1   Service user involvement activities log.

- Will any of the information collected be confidential, personal or sensitive? If so, how will this information be handled and stored?
- How will the information be reported on, for example will it be incorporated into a final research report or conference presentation?

In the context of critical review, guidelines have been created for assessing the quality and impact of service user involvement in published papers and grant applications (Wright et al. 2010). The appraisal guidelines were developed on the basis of available literature and experiences from studies involving cancer patients and carers in the design and conduct of research. Nine appraisal criteria were developed, including issues such as: 'Is the rationale for involving users clearly demonstrated?', 'Is the level of service user involvement appropriate?', 'Is the recruitment strategy appropriate?', and 'Is the nature of training appropriate?'

Using reflective techniques

To critically examine issues about the quality of involvement processes, service users and researchers can make use of a range of reflective techniques. Most qualitative researchers will be familiar with the idea of maintaining a research diary. Reflective writing is perhaps the most commonly used reflective technique. Other methods include interactive methods within groups, perspective taking such as reflective interviews with those who have participated in a study, and creative representations and conceptual diagrams (Eppler 2006). Figure 9.2 illustrates these and some other reflective techniques

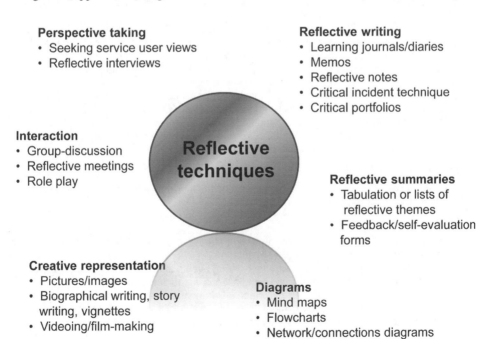

Perspective taking
- Seeking service user views
- Reflective interviews

Reflective writing
- Learning journals/diaries
- Memos
- Reflective notes
- Critical incident technique
- Critical portfolios

Interaction
- Group-discussion
- Reflective meetings
- Role play

Reflective techniques

Reflective summaries
- Tabulation or lists of reflective themes
- Feedback/self-evaluation forms

Creative representation
- Pictures/images
- Biographical writing, story writing, vignettes
- Videoing/film-making

Diagrams
- Mind maps
- Flowcharts
- Network/connections diagrams

Figure 9.2   Reflective techniques.

Box 9.2   Evaluating young people's experiences of involvement

Case study

CLIC Sargent – The UK's leading cancer charity for children

Jane Coad, Professor in Children and Family Nursing, Coventry University, Alisha Newman, Participation Manager Children & Young People, Dr Bernie Carter, Professor of Children's Nursing University of Central Lancashire, Joanna Smith, Research Fellow, University of the West of England, Andrew Moore, Research Associate University of Central Lancashire, Dr Zoe Lee, CLIC Sargent Volunteer & Research Associate, and Andrew Cooper, Head of Services, CLIC Sargent.

Exploring new models of care with young people

CLIC Sargent was commissioned to carry out the study by the Children & Young People's Work Stream as part of the National Cancer Survivorship Initiative. CLIC Sargent together with ten test communities was funded by the Department of Health to explore new models and approaches of care for children and young people living with and beyond cancer. Alongside the main consultation study, CLIC Sargent commissioned an evaluation study to find out about the children's perspectives and opinions about taking part in the activities during the workshops.

Cancer survivors aged 7–13 living in England were invited to tell CLIC Sargent about the impact of cancer on their world. The children were given the option of giving their views at an activity afternoon held at six venues nationally. The afternoon used children's arts-based activities to gather rich quality narrative. Children's postal activity packs combined written and illustrated contributions from children living with and beyond cancer. Children and families were very supportive of the study, and a total of 90 children took part. In total 49 children attended an activity afternoon and 41 children returned a completed postal activity pack. The study gathered rich quality narrative which combined written and illustrated contributions from children living with and beyond cancer. The full report can be downloaded at www.clicsargent.org.uk.

The method used to consult children at the activity afternoons was independently evaluated (1). The evaluation team included four researchers who took detailed narrative field notes recording impressions, quotations and details of the children whom they were observing. Arts-based activities and participant observation were used as they allowed the evaluation team to respond to the children and facilitators where necessary, but not to become overtly involved in the running or processes of the consultation activities. The aims of the evaluation study were to (1) evaluate the children's experiences and perceptions of both the approach and participatory methods used for the main CLIC Sargent study; (2) identify, evaluate and report any issues following each event which could potentially improve subsequent consultation exercises.

Issues to be aware of:

- In this study the children felt that the activities were 'fun' and 'brilliant' but the evaluation helped to identify ways of improving involvement.

Helpful ideas:

- The activities in the workshop were an hour in duration, which children told us was too long. The activities need to be shorter in duration.
- It is important to include some 'down time' during events to let children have fun and let off some steam. For example, playing with balloons is safe and energetic.
- Activities need to be accessible but older children may need to be challenged and stretched more to keep them interested. Encourage active participation by using movement and games or prompts like photographs to stimulate interest.

- Children may be able to relate more to a research activity if they are invited to write a letter to a person they know or a celebrity they admire.
- Timing the coordinated finish of activities creates challenges. Facilitators need to have some activities available with which to engage the children if their group finishes early.
- Researchers who are experienced group facilitators and comfortable with using arts-based activities are essential to ensuring the smooth running of workshops. It is difficult to adequately prepare facilitators on the day of the event. Facilitator training could be enhanced by using a demonstration video.
- Venues, food and refreshments all need to be child-friendly. Rooms need to have plenty of light and be an appropriate size.
- The size of the group influences the dynamics of how children interact. Age range and mix of abilities and needs are also important considerations. Ensure that everyone in the group is able to join in and enjoy the same things.

that researchers and service users can make use of to enhance the quality of the research and their own practices.

Some issues to consider when deciding which reflective techniques to use are:

- Who will be asked to reflect on their experiences; service users, researchers or everyone involved in the research?
- How will reflection be explained to those who are being asked to reflect? What might their preferences and concerns be?
- What types of issues will people be asked to reflect on, for example their personal experiences of involvement or the research topic or issues raised during the research?
- Will people be asked just to comment on their experiences or to make suggestions for how things could have been done better?
- Will you use individual reflective methods or group reflection (consider the different advantages of confidential feedback versus open discussion)?
- Will reflection be attributed to individuals or will it be anonymous? Will everyone see what has been said or will a summary be written about general comments and suggestions?
- How will you deal with any negative experiences or feedback?

In the case study (Box 9.2), young people involved in the work of the CLIC Sargent charity were asked to reflect on their experiences of taking part in different cancer research activities. The evaluation made use of interactive methods – an activity afternoon – as well as the option of postal activity packs for children who could not attend in person. In this evaluation, the young people were able to provide detailed comments about the timing and duration of activities. They also made suggestions about incorporating play and movement into the research work to make it more interesting. In this example, the researchers were able to draw on their skills in facilitation and the use of arts-based activities to elicit young people's experiences.

Reflexivity and service user involvement

Reflexivity is an ongoing process which is often used in nursing and healthcare research to reflect on the different factors that influence research processes and outcomes (Carolan 2003). It can be used to examine any research study or programme from the perspective of those that are involved in it as the work progresses. Ongoing reflexivity can be more advantageous than waiting until the end of a study to undertake a one-off evaluation because it means there is the opportunity to make improvements during the research. Healthcare practitioners may be familiar with using reflective practice as part of their professional development work. In a similar way to reflective practice, reflexivity can lead to continuous improvements in research processes and outcomes because it encourages research teams to examine the strengths and limitations of what they are doing in a methodological way (Alvesson and Sköldberg 2000). Reflexivity can support learning and professional development by exploring personal understandings and perspectives (Dowling 2006). Service users can also benefit from being involved in using reflexivity because it helps to structure lines of thinking and reflection about the research and personal involvement. This section introduces four different types of reflexivity and explains how they can be used to improve the quality of service user involvement in research.

Self-critical reflexivity → Personal thoughts and actions

Self-critical reflection, or personal reflection, means reflecting on your own thoughts and actions. It could involve recording one's own perceptions, judgements, reactions and behaviours in relation to an issue or practice (Finlay and Gough 2003). The purpose of self-critical reflection is to examine how factors such as past experience, feelings, mood, personal agendas and aspirations, influence research processes. In relation to service user involvement self-critical reflection can help to examine why individual people are interested in a particular issue or topic and what they may be able to contribute to the research. It can also help to uncover why certain people feel strongly about certain issues and the types of insights they might be able to share. Self-critical reflexivity acknowledges that everyone has a different background and set of personal experiences which influence their understanding and approach to the research. For example, people with professional backgrounds are likely to draw on the types of disciplinary language and concepts that they have become familiar with to approach research questions from the perspective of a healthcare professional. On the other hand, service users are likely to draw on their personal experiences of health and illness and tend to see things from the patient's perspective.

Interpersonal reflexivity → Interactions with others

Interpersonal reflexivity means paying attention to the relationships that influence any research study or programme. This could include looking at interactions between the people that are undertaking the research. It could also include looking at the relationships which led to the undertaking of a particular research activity, such as the establishment of a research partnership between individuals in different organisations. Examining interpersonal interactions can help to reveal the established norms surrounding a given practice. In the case of service user involvement, interpersonal reflexivity could help to reveal expectations about who will take on certain roles in the research. It may be that some researchers and service users interact well in some aspects of the research but not so well in other areas. Reflecting on such issues can help to establish good working practices throughout the whole research study.

Contextual reflexivity → Concepts, theory and methods

Contextual reflexivity involves examining how established concepts, theories and methods inform and influence practice (Johns 2004). In relation to nursing and healthcare research it could mean questioning the types of research methods and techniques that are used in any study rather than other methods. Contextual reflexivity leads to the question: How might things have been done differently if an alternative frame of reference or way of thinking had been used? Examples could be how the use of different concepts of quality of life, well-being or patient experience influences the research.

Critical reflexivity → Political, ethical and social contexts

Critical reflexivity is concerned with issues of power, which enter into all research activities. It involves making explicit any ethical, political or social issues encountered and the impact this may have had on the people involved, or those not involved (Mauthner and Doucet 2003). Critical reflexivity involves asking what questions, issues or ways of thinking have been privileged by whom and for what reasons? In relation to service user involvement in research, critical reflexivity can help to explore how the research may help to empower certain individuals, for example but providing patients with better information about their condition or better treatment or care.

The reflexivity framework presented in Figure 9.3 can help research teams to find a balance between the four types of reflexivity described above (Smith 2011). It could help researchers and service users to put their decisions and actions into perspective and assess favoured lines of knowledge and practice.

The remaining sections of this chapter focus in more detail on two specific perspectives of quality in service user involvement – experiences of involvement and building quality research environments to support involvement.

Quality experiences of involvement

This section of the chapter looks at how research teams can work towards quality experiences of involvement. Here, quality is approached from the perspectives of those that are involved in the research, which could mean both service users and researchers. Three areas of personal experience – ability, potential and sense of being – have been identified

Self-critical (reflecting on your own thoughts and actions)	Interpersonal (reflecting on interactions with others)
Key considerations could include:	Key considerations could include:
• Why are you interested in a particular issue or topic? • What questions seem important to you? • What informs your views? • What aspects of your background are you drawing on? • What personal experience do you have?	• What disciplinary-based ideas and frameworks inform your interpretations? • What aspects of your disciplinary background lead you to dwell on certain aspects of an issue or problem and not others? • Whose perspectives might be missing or overlooked?
Contextual (reflecting on concepts, theories or methods used)	Critical (reflecting on political, ethical and social context)
Key considerations could include:	Key considerations could include:
• What insights were generated, or do you hope to generate, by using a particular approach to the research? • On what basis do/will these insights contribute to knowledge or practice? • What different insights may be/have been made if a different approach or perspective had been taken?	• What is the political context in this situation, what are the contentious issues? • Is there a political agenda at stake: what might the outcomes be? • Who might gain because of what has been done or not done: who might lose out?

Figure 9.3   Types of reflexivity.

as contributing to quality experiences of service user involvement (Morrow et al. 2010). Here these are presented as prompts for researchers and service users to explore their own opinions and experiences about what quality involvement means to them. Key themes for personal reflection are illustrated by Figure 9.4. It can be useful to spend time considering such views as the research progresses so that research teams can work towards maximising everyone's personal contributions. This should not be thought of as a checklist of items that researchers or service users should do; they are meant to encourage reflection and learning about service user involvement.

Ability

In terms of being able to participate in research, much attention has been given to practical issues such as payments for expenses and fees for service user's time. As explained in Chapter 3, good practice guidance on payments is now available ('Payments' section). A wider issue is whether service users and researchers are able to access sufficient research resources, for example to meet the cost of funding language translators. A further issue in relation to this theme is the extent to which service users feel they are able to contribute and achieve their own goals by being involved in the work of mainstream research institutions. A related issue is whether service users feel able to make decisions about how to plan and undertake the research or to select the techniques and methods that

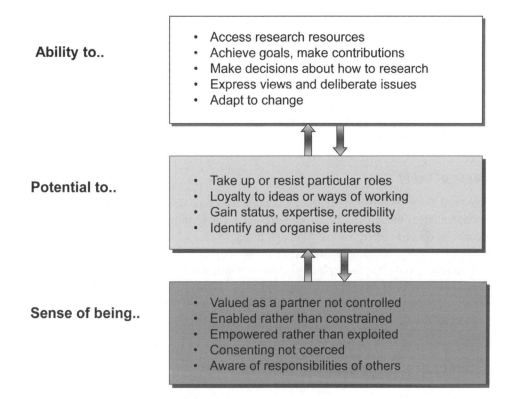

Ability to..

- Access research resources
- Achieve goals, make contributions
- Make decisions about how to research
- Express views and deliberate issues
- Adapt to change

Potential to..

- Take up or resist particular roles
- Loyalty to ideas or ways of working
- Gain status, expertise, credibility
- Identify and organise interests

Sense of being..

- Valued as a partner not controlled
- Enabled rather than constrained
- Empowered rather than exploited
- Consenting not coerced
- Aware of responsibilities of others

Figure 9.4   Key themes for reflection – Personal involvement.

might be used. For example, service users often have direct experience of the issues under consideration but they may not be able to translate these into agenda items, discussion points, arguments, research questions and so on. A further aspect of personal ability is the ability to adapt to new situations and circumstances.

Potential

Under the theme of personal potential is the issue of roles. Decisions made early on in the research can have a significant impact on the potential for involvement. In most cases, opportunities for service user involvement are shaped at proposal stage by a researcher's expectations of how such relationships might operate and the type of role service users might take on. Some researchers may perceive service user's views as data within the research or see themselves as an intermediary between service users and the research process. Others may see service users as collaborators, stakeholders, partners or co-researchers depending on the context of the research. Proposal development is recognised as being a key area where service users could be more involved in exploring the types of ideas and insights that they might bring to the work. Seeking to understand such factors from the start may help to establish realistic expectations about what can be achieved and to devise ways of working that as far as possible align with what service users want from their involvement. Personal potential is also linked to the types of professional credentials and experience that are valued within research systems. For some service users potential could include the opportunity to gain recognised status as research partners, expertise in research methods or credibility as independent user researchers. As recognised members of a research institution, service users may have greater opportunity to identify and organise their research ideas and values leading to a positive experience of involvement.

Sense of being

The third theme of personal experience is sense of being. This theme encompasses ideas about feeling as though you are an active research partner rather than controlled by other people involved in the research. Although different people will have different expectations about who should take charge, set the agenda, or report on the research, ideally everyone involved in the research should feel enabled rather than constrained. Furthermore, they should feel empowered rather than exploited. What is important is that everyone is aware of the types of roles and responsibilities each person is taking on and that they are willing to do so.

Quality environments for involvement

In this section, three further themes are presented to expand thinking about quality beyond the actions of individual service users or researchers. These themes are: research relationships, ways of doing research and research structures (see Figure 9.5). By considering these themes and drawing attention to quality at an organisational and research systems level, research teams may be more able to recognise and challenge any barriers to involvement. Taking time to reflect on service user involvement could help organisations to:

• Balance competing pressures and priorities
• Meet national policies for service user involvement
• Expand the role and function of service users
• Link work and people across research communities and institutions
• Understand circumstances of non-engagement or disengagement
• Create welcoming and comfortable environments for service users
• Establish systems, for example for training or payments
• Develop protocols and best practice guidance

Discussing some of these issues in a real-life situation requires sensitivity and skills that may necessitate facilitation from someone outside of the immediate research team or organisation. The aims of honest reflection and quality improvement should be emphasised to avoid unhelpful criticism or defensiveness. In some cases it may work better to draw on

Research relationships	• Requirements and incentives • Funding opportunities • Information about involvement • Expectations and prevailing conditions • Communication structures • Outcomes which are awarded value
Ways of doing research	• Roles available to be taken up • Criteria and responsibilities • Established research practices • Research methods and techniques
Research structures	• Institutions and programmes • Ethics and governance systems • Methods and techniques of research • Research technologies, monitoring and reporting systems

Figure 9.5   Key themes for reflection – Research context.

the themes to create a written list of issues that people can reflect on individually in their own time. Other teams may wish to simply use these tools as prompts to structure their thinking, or to inform reports or publications about service user involvement. User research-ers and user-led research organisations could also make use of these prompts to self-assess their own processes and improve ways of working.

Research relationships

There are multiple types of requirements and incentives for service user involvement in research. If service users do not feel researchers have the right reasons for wanting to involve them, they may feel their involvement is tokenistic (as discussed in Chapter 2). At the same time researchers may be under pressure to find resources and support for service user involvement alongside working to meet project deadlines and deliver research outputs (Staniszewska et al. 2007). From the researcher's perspective, explaining the types of goals that they want from the research may help to clarify different perspectives of how best service users may contribute. Many previous authors have argued that quality involvement requires adequate funding opportunities – in particular, support for additional researcher time. Researchers need to have time to put together information for service users about the research and about how they could be involved. There also needs to be enough time for two-way communication throughout the research. Without investing time in developing relationships researchers may not be able to attend to, may not listen to, or may not 'hear' suggestions articulated by service users. At worst it could lead to a situation where topics for research studies are selected and defined by professional groups without any possibility for the consideration of service user perspectives. As a result, service users may choose not to engage in studies where they feel they will have little say in or over the research. Understanding quality also means exploring the dynamic qualities of research relationships within the prevailing conditions of research environments. Such factors could include changes in expectations, different intentions and goals, and alternative perspectives of successes and achievements. There is also a need to better understand how organisational communication structures help or hinder service user involvement in research. A further area for consideration is the relationship between quality service user involvement and the types of outcomes which are awarded value within research organisations and systems (as discussed in the next chapter).

Ways of doing the research

Quality involvement could mean having a clear role in a research relationship and clarity about the types of skills and experiences being contributed. Again, these are issues that require time for exploration and review. Different research institutions will have better developed roles for service users than others and there is much to be learnt from mental health and social care research. Nursing and healthcare research could work towards better defined criteria and responsibilities for service user roles. Being an active participant in research requires learning about established research practices. Service user involvement is not guaranteed to be safe, legitimate, or productive. There is always the possibility that involvement processes can become unethical or illegal. Although these negative outcomes could be fully unintentional, there need to be safety nets in place within organisations and research systems to protect researchers, service users and participants in the research. Reflecting on ways of doing research may help to develop research methods and techniques that help to limit risk and improve the quality of research outcomes.

Research structures

Quality involvement also means raising questions about whether involvement is supported or hindered by research structures. It involves asking questions such as whether involvement is valued and assessed as part of the work of the organisation, whether it is supported by existing ethical and governance systems and linked into research structures and networks. Research teams might also ask how service user involvement works alongside the methods and techniques of the research. There is also the issue of how to make sure that involvement work is reported on in the mainstream research literature (see 'Reporting Impact', Chapter 10). At the present time, it is largely down to research teams to choose to provide explanations and describe outcomes of service user involvement when publishing the research.

> **Key principles for practice**
>
> - Right from the start research teams should follow principles for successful involvement. These are: documenting the roles of service users in the research, maintaining financial records of funding and payments, reporting and acknowledging service user contributions in research reports and papers, meeting training needs, seeking service user's advice about recruitment and participant information, and disseminating research findings to service users and relevant service user groups in appropriate formats and easily understandable language.
> - Research teams can demonstrate active and direct participation of service users in the commissioning, design, undertaking or evaluation of research by keeping an activities log about what happens through the research and reporting on involvement at the end of a study or programme.
> - Service users and researchers can make use of a range of reflective techniques to examine issues about the quality of involvement processes such as reflective diaries, feedback and evaluation forms, or reflective interviewing.
> - Research teams can make use of reflexivity to pay attention to the personal, interpersonal, contextual, political and ethical factors which influence research. Reflexivity can help to identify the strengths and limitations of what has been done and make decisions behind the research more explicit.
> - Research teams can work towards quality experiences of involvement by understanding the perspectives of those that are involved in the research. Three areas of personal experience – ability, potential and sense of being – can be used as prompts for reflection and learning.
> - By considering quality at an organisational and research systems level, research teams may be more able to build more supportive research environments and to challenge any barriers to involvement.

References

Alvesson, M. and Sköldberg, K. (2000) *Reflexive Methodology: New Vistas for Qualitative Research*. London: Sage Publications.

Blackburn, H., Hanley, B., and Staley, K. (2010) *Turning the pyramid upside down: examples of public involvement in social care research*. Eastleigh: INVOLVE.

Carolan, M. (2003) Reflexivity: a personal journal during data collection. *Nurse Researcher*, 10 (3): 7–14.

Dowling, M. (2006) Approaches to reflexivity in qualitative research. *Nurse Researcher*, 13 (3): 7–21.

Eppler, M. (2006) A comparison between concept maps, mind maps, conceptual diagrams, and visual metaphors as complementary tools for knowledge construction and sharing. *Information Visualization*, 5: 3.

Finlay, L. and Gough, B. (eds) (2003) *Reflexivity. A Practical Guide for Researchers in Health and Social Sciences*. Oxford: Blackwell.

Johns, C. (2004) *Becoming a Reflective Practitioner*, 2nd edn. Oxford: Blackwell.

Mauthner, N. and Doucet, A. (2003) Reflexive accounts and accounts of reflexivity in qualitative data analysis. *Sociology*, 37: 413–43.

Morrow, E., Ross, F., Grocott, P., and Bennett, J. (2010) A model and measure of quality service user involvement in health research. Special Issue of *International Journal of Consumer Studies*, 34 (5): 532–9.

Schrank, B. and Wallcraft, J. (2009) Good practice guidance. In: Wallcraft, J., Schrank, B., and Amering, M. (eds) *Handbook of Service User Involvement in Mental Health Research*. Chichester: Wiley-Blackwell.

Smith, E. (2011) Teaching critical reflection. *Teaching in Higher Education*, 16 (2): 211–23.

Staniszewska, S., Jones, N., Newburn, M., and Marshall, S. (2007) User involvement in the development of a research bid: barriers, enablers and impacts. *Health Expectations*, 10 (2): 173–83.

Telford, R., Boote, J., and Cooper, C. (2004) What does it mean to involve consumers successfully in NHS research? A consensus study. *Health Expectations*, 7 (3): 209–20.

Wright, D., Foster, C., Amir, Z., Elliott, J., and Wilson, R. (2010) Critical appraisal guidelines for assessing the quality and impact of user involvement in research. *Health Expectations*, 13 (4): 359–68.

Chapter 10

Impact

Key summary points

- *Why we need to know about impact*: Building an evidence base for service user involvement in research is important because it will help to: show whether it is effective, demonstrate the benefits and drawbacks, understand the best approaches to service user involvement in research, reflect and learn from the evidence, inform policy development and support strategies, and identify what future research needs to be done.
- *Designing an assessment*: When undertaking an assessment of impact it is important to be clear about your conceptual understanding of the relationship between what is being assessed, research, policy and practice. Service users can be involved in clarifying the priorities, purposes and perspectives of the assessment.
- *Recognising impact*: There are many different types of research impact. Before mapping the impacts of interest, it is helpful to be clear about your conceptual understanding of the relationship between service user involvement and service development and improvement as this will help to define the scope and boundaries of the assessment of impact.
- *Recording impact*: Any assessment of impact needs to be underpinned by a good quality monitoring system designed to capture impacts as they occur. Most impact studies use a mixed method approach. It is also useful to consider whether service users can be involved in the impact assessment process.
- *Reporting impact*: As with other research and evaluation, the results of impact studies should be made available in a variety of formats (summaries, reports, presentations, web material). As few impact studies of service user involvement have been published, efforts should be made to put the findings into the public domain. It is helpful to consider at the start of the process how you might deal with challenging findings, such as limited evidence of impact, to maximise individual and organisational learning.

Handbook of Service User Involvement in Nursing and Healthcare Research, First Edition.
Elizabeth Morrow, Annette Boaz, Sally Brearley and Fiona Ross.
© 2012 Elizabeth Morrow, Annette Boaz, Sally Brearley and Fiona Ross.
Published 2012 by Blackwell Publishing Ltd.

Why we need to know about impact

Demonstrating impact is an issue that faces anyone who is working to engage, promote or understand service user involvement in health services and health research (Staniszewska 2009). It is also an issue that public services and social care researchers have been concerned with for some time (Baxter et al. 2001). In this chapter we explore the different ways in which impact is assessed and the rationales that underpin impact assessment.

There are a number of different rationales for assessing the impact of any activity or intervention. These include encouraging learning, audit and accountability, promoting individual and organisational achievements and demonstrating effectiveness. It is helpful to be clear about which of these rationales applies to you when embarking upon an impact assessment, bearing in mind that there may be more than one purpose, for example to show effectiveness and to capture learning across a programme of research.

Many researchers and service users strongly believe that active involvement in the research process leads to research that is more relevant to people and is more likely to be used. The argument is that research which takes on board the views and perspectives of the public is more likely to produce results that can be used to improve practice in nursing and health care (Entwistle et al. 1998). Furthermore, research findings may be viewed as more credible when they are informed by service user perspectives (Boote et al. 2010).

As we saw in Chapter 1, service user involvement is often thought of as being ethical and that people who are affected by research should have a right to have a say in what and how research is undertaken. For them, they may feel there is no need to prove or justify its impact because it is the morally right thing to do. Involving service users can also help to improve research practice and the experience of participants in the research. For example, the information sheet given to potential participants may be written in more accessible language that better explains what they are being asked to do. Service user involvement can also inform good practice in access issues such as timing and location for interviewing and meetings. In the context of clinical trials for breast cancer prevention service users helped to identify ways in which they could strengthen the research (Psillidis et al. 1997).

A further argument is that being involved in research can have significant personal benefits for service users who are involved, which could be considered as one form of impact. In nursing and midwifery research there are accounts from both service users and researchers about the types of benefits they have experienced, such as improved understanding of the issues under investigation, therapeutic benefits (Peddie et al. 2006), more confidence, skills and greater opportunity for social interaction and personal development (Smith et al. 2008).

At the present time we do not have a strong evidence base to demonstrate that service user involvement is making a difference, or to communicate to others that it is worthwhile and has more benefits than drawbacks (Boote et al. 2002). There is a need to further develop an evidence base for service user involvement in research (INVOLVE 2009) because this will help to:

- Assess the impact(s) of service user involvement in research
- Demonstrate the benefits and drawbacks of service user involvement in research
- Understand the best approaches to service user involvement in research
- Reflect and learn from the evidence
- Inform policy development and support strategies
- Identify what future research needs to be done

Designing an assessment of impact

Although service user involvement is increasingly accepted as good practice across health and social care research, it is nevertheless widely acknowledged that there is a need to show impact, as described above. This is part of a wider interest by research funders in assessing the impact of research (Cooksey 2006; UK Evaluation Forum 2006). Research impact assessment is considered to be a challenging area of evaluation practice (Nutley et al. 2007) and there are specific problems in evaluating the impact of service user involvement, discussed in the next section. In general, there are issues of:

- Attribution: How do we know whether the research led to the impacts identified?
- Timing: When might impact be expected to occur?
- Capturing context: What types of external factors and local issues are important influences?
- Capturing complexity: How do all the factors, issues and interactions interrelate and to what effect?
- Focus: Whether to track impact forwards from research studies or backwards from evidence that informed decisions in policy or practice.

A range of tools and techniques have been developed to assess research impact more widely (Hanney et al. 2007; Boaz et al. 2009), which can be applied to better understand the impact of service user involvement in research. We will briefly discuss some of the thinking in this field. When undertaking an assessment of impact it is beneficial to be clear about your conceptual understanding of the relationship between what is being assessed and research, policy and practice. As illustrated by Figure 10.1, a good assessment will consider the priorities, purposes and perspectives that are informing the aims and process. It could be beneficial to use this structure to clarify why an assessment is being undertaken.

Another approach to clarifying the aims of the assessment is to develop a Theories of Change sequence chain (Connell and Kubisch 1998). This involves writing down a list of service user activities, intended outputs and outcomes (early, intermediate through to long-term). These can be discussed with colleagues and other stakeholders to clarify the role and meaning of service user involvement in the context being studied. The sequence chain can then inform the approach to assessment and the methods used. Developing a Theories of Change sequence chain is not dissimilar to setting the aims and objectives for a project at the outset of an evaluation.

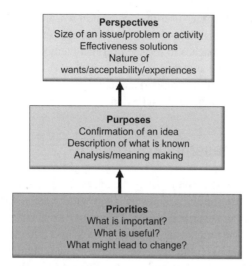

Figure 10.1   Building an evidence base.

It is also helpful to consider, right at the start of the process, the ways in which service users and other key stakeholders such as policymakers and healthcare practitioners might be involved in the impact assessment process. For example, these groups could be invited to discuss the priorities, purposes and perspectives of the assessment or to help develop a Theories of Change sequence chain to guide the assessment. It is also important to remember that for some people focusing on issues about the impact of service user involvement could be perceived as undermining the argument that involving service users is morally right and of intrinsic value.

Recognising impact

Before considering methods for recording the impact, it is important to note a number of issues relating to service user involvement as an intervention (Staniszewska et al. 2008):

- Service user involvement takes many forms ranging from consultation of service users at particular stages of the research process to research led and/or controlled by users.
- Service user involvement might be a one-off or an ongoing activity.
- Little attention has been paid to identifying negative and unintended impacts of service user involvement.
- Service user involvement is a complex intervention; it is problematic to try to test it under randomised or controlled conditions.

Figure 10.2 lists some key ideas about evaluating service user involvement. This advice is adapted from the Medical Research Council's guidelines for complex evaluation. Bearing these issues in mind there are a number of ways in which we can begin to examine the impact of service user involvement in research. As always, there is more than one way of

> ➢ A good theoretical understanding is needed of how service user involvement may cause change – a range of impacts should be considered
>
> ➢ Lack of impact may reflect early development stages rather than no actual impact – a process evaluation can help to identify issues about where things are working well and may lead to impact
>
> ➢ Impact at a project level is likely to reflect higher level processes such as funding or support – looking across projects can help to take into account wider issues that affect service user involvement
>
> ➢ Focusing on one type of outcome may not adequately reflect what has happened – a range of measures will be needed and unintended consequences picked up where possible
>
> ➢ Trying to standardize involvement in order to measure it is inappropriate – service user involvement works better where it is adapted to local settings and projects

Figure 10.2   Key ideas for evaluating service user involvement.

approaching the issues. For example, we might ask what difference service user involvement makes on a number of levels – to the individual people involved, to the research, or to society. Any assessment of impact needs to take into consideration contextual issues, such as the different people involved in commissioning, carrying out, receiving and responding to the results of research. We might also be interested in looking at the impact of the process or the outcomes of the research.

For these reasons it can be more useful to think of impact as a set of issues, rather than a single measure, outcome or value. Identifying what the impact has been could involve looking at a range of outcomes from a range of different perspectives. Outcomes might include how decisions about the research have been made and the influence it has had. Different perspectives might include not only the views of researchers or service users involved but also the types of impact that commissioners, policymakers or other key stakeholders are interested in and likely to be able to act upon.

Many researchers are primarily concerned with the quality and rigour of research and whether service user involvement might improve or compromise the research results. At the same time, researchers who have worked with service users often believe that their involvement has led to benefits because of bringing the work into perspective – that of the people most closely affected by it. Box 10.1 draws on a discussion paper produced by a working group of researchers and service users in the UK (INVOLVE 2007) who have come together to identify some of the ways in which the research might be influenced by service users.

In the UK, research has been undertaken to investigate whether it is feasible to evaluate the impact of public involvement on health and social care research (Barber et al. 2011). The research study used mixed methods including a two-round Delphi study (a consensus reaching exercise) with pre-specified 80% consensus criterion. Follow-up interviews

---

Box 10.1   How the research may be influenced by service users

(a) *The nature of the research questions*: Both the broad research question and the more specific questions asked may become more relevant to those most directly influenced by the research.

(b) *The choice of research tools (e.g. questionnaires, outcome measures)*: The tools chosen may measure outcomes, ask questions or seek understanding about what is of concern or relevance to service users.

(c) *The relevance of research outcomes*: As a result of the above, the outcomes of the research may be more meaningful, not just to service users or carers, but also to the practitioners or people expected to implement the research results.

(d) *Data collection, analysis and interpretation*: Where service users or carers are involved in data collection and analysis and interpretation, for example from interviews with peers, the quality of these processes can be improved. There is some evidence that more open and honest responses are given where interviewees perceive their interviewer to be a peer.

(e) *Commissioning process*: Involvement in the generation of research topics for funding, short-listing/selection of successful applications, candidate interviewing and subsequent research management are all processes that can benefit from a service user perspective.

(f) *The experience of being a research participant*: Active public involvement in the planning, design and data collection of research can help to improve the experience of those taking part in research and facilitate recruitment. It can influence the way the research is carried out, how participants are treated and the quality of the information that is provided.

---

were conducted with a purposive sample of 14 panellists. UK and international panellists came from different settings, including universities, health and social care institutions and charitable organisations. They comprised a total of 124 researchers, members of the public, research managers, research commissioners and policymakers. Many panellists highlighted the importance of evaluating the impact of public involvement (109 of 145 panellists, 75.2% in the first round of the Delphi process), while acknowledging the complexity of the process. Consensus was reached that it is feasible to evaluate the impact of public involvement on five of 16 impact issues. These were:

- Identifying topics to be researched
- Prioritising topics to be researched
- Disseminating research
- Members of the public involved in the research
- Members of the research team

Interestingly, the highest level of consensus related to the feasibility of evaluating the impact of public involvement on members of the public involved in research, information which could help to secure commitment to involvement in the future (an area of impact discussed further in Chapter 12: Conclusions). The research also revealed areas of public involvement in research that panellists felt could not be feasibly evaluated. A further 11 of the 16 impact issues examined were not considered feasible to evaluate according to the consensus criterion set (80% consensus). These were:

- Commissioning research
- Research design
- Managing research
- Collecting data
- Analysing research findings
- Interpreting research findings
- Determining the usefulness of research findings
- Implementing research findings
- The overall quality of public involvement in a research study or research-related activity
- The overall quality of the research
- The overall impact of the research

Reasons put forward included the high costs of evaluation and reservations about the feasibility of evaluating the impact of public involvement on research design in basic science. Other reservations reflect the difficulties of defining and assessing quality in research and impact of research (see Chapter 9).

So we are building up a picture of impact as a complex idea in itself. In the context of service user involvement in nursing and healthcare research assessing impact is not likely to work by comparing similar research carried out with and without service user involvement in order to see how the outcomes are different, such as in a comparative research study. This is because there are too many variables involved to make such a comparison valid. It is unlikely that replication or controlled methods would be useful or achievable because service user involvement is not a controllable intervention. Service user involvement is characterised by dynamic interactions and sometimes unexpected outcomes. An alternative way of assessing impact might be to ask a number of questions about the usefulness of the research and its outcomes from the perspective of different stakeholders.

One test for the usefulness of research is whether or not it has practical application and if it has led to change. There is emerging evidence in some fields that service user involvement in research improves the relevance of research and therefore is more likely to lead to implementation of new knowledge or to change things for the better (Staniszewska et al. 2008). The case study (Box 10.2), assessing the benefits of service user involvement in health research from the Warwick Diabetes Care Research User Group, provides an insight into the complexities of assessment of impact.

Recording impact

The impacts of service user involvement are often lost due to poor systems for recording relevant activities. Therefore, a first step towards capturing impact is to put in place a monitoring system. As described in Chapter 9, reflective tools can be as basic as a paper impact diary or as complex as a computer-based system for recording, for example number of events, number of attendees at meetings, results from feedback forms and so on (see 'Using reflective techniques' section). It could be helpful to consider the types of information that might be captured by a monitoring system (Figure 10.3). Once a

Box 10.2   Assessing the benefits of service user involvement

Case study

Antje Lindenmeyer, Senior Research Fellow, Warwick Diabetes Care Research and Education User Group

The Warwick Diabetes Research and Education User Group is a group of lay people who have an active interest in the experiences and care of people living with diabetes. Since 2001, the group has been involved in all aspects of diabetes research conducted by the Warwick Diabetes Research Team. Group meetings are held bi-monthly, but quite often 'focus' groups are formed to deal with a specific piece of work. Some members also engage with the group's activities from home. From time to time the group mounts training events so that its members can increase their skills in assisting with research projects using varied research designs and methods.

'How do we know whether service user involvement in diabetes research is effective or meaningful'?

For our qualitative study of researchers' and users' real life experience of involvement, we conducted semi-structured interviews with researchers who had worked extensively with the group and discussions at the regular user group meetings. Interviews and discussions focused on what difference consultation with users had made to research projects, and what had made the group more or less effective in improving research.
  We found that:

- Both researchers and users felt that the group's involvement resulted in more funded research that was relevant to the experience and requirements of service users.
- The service users brought to the group their practical experience of living with diabetes and a connection to the world in which the research would be used.
- The fact that the group had been established for some time allowed for users to have a more detailed understanding of the research process, for relationships with the researchers to develop and a collaborative research ethos to form.
- A partial shift of power from researchers to users occurred as the group was chaired by a lay member and researchers were in the minority.

Key issues to be aware of:

- It was extremely hard to evaluate the impact of service user involvement. Paradoxically, the more users and researchers worked as peers on specific projects, the more difficult it became to show impact as involvement was informal or as part of joint research meetings.
- It is important to stress that the group should not be considered to be representative of the patient population or participants of future trials.
- Building a group of this nature will take years but our experience is that close collaboration between researchers and users in the long-term improved research.

Helpful ideas:

- Qualitative methods were particularly helpful in capturing the personal interactions between researchers and service users and their understandings of meaningful research.

monitoring system is in place it is possible to consider conducting more in-depth research to capture impact based on trends or issues that are detected.

Impact assessments are typically mixed-method studies. This means the methods used to assess impact are diverse and can be qualitative or quantitative approaches. A recent review (Boaz et al. 2009) on impact assessment approaches summarised the different methods used as:

Key information it can be useful to record:

Date/time: At what stage in the project/programme is the record being made?
Type of impact: What is the type of impact observed?
Who is involved: Who are the key individuals and groups that are involved on this occasion?
Who is the impact affecting: Service users, researchers, participants in the study, other people outside of the research team such as practitioners or policymakers, the public generally?
Setting: Where is the impact being felt/made, e.g. in the organisation/outside of the organisations
Mechanisms: How is influence being made, what are the mechanisms? e.g. communication, meetings, information resources, use of evidence,
Context: What other factors could be having an impact? e.g. political issues, resource issues, decisions that have been made, people's opinions or experiences
Key points of interest: What implications might there be for policy or practice?

Figure 10.3 Identifying and recording impact.

- Qualitative methods including semi-structured interviews, documentary analysis, field visits and observations
- Quantitative methods including surveys, bibliometrics and patent/new technology tracking
- Panels and peer review
- Workshops and focus groups
- Process tracking including historical tracing, positive utilisation narratives and impact logs
- Literature review
- Network mapping and analysis

Choosing methods for an impact study will depend on a variety of questions, starting with which evaluation methods might be used to explore the outcomes of interest to those involved in the project. For example, the success of service user/researcher/policy networks might be explored using network mapping, while an analysis of responsiveness of research to policy needs might use interviews with policymakers, and documentary analysis. And, in the case of involving service users in agenda setting, an impact study might involve interviews with stakeholders, documentary analysis or workshops. It is also useful to think about which methods are credible in the field in which the impact assessment occurs. For example, if numbers are considered persuasive, as they are in most areas of healthcare research, then it might be worth considering ways in which quantitative data can be collected or used to 'back up' other types of qualitative data.

One of the key challenges with gathering convincing evidence of impact is the problem of attribution. This means asking to what extent are the impacts identified attributable to service user involvement rather than another factor. Attribution becomes harder if the researcher is keen to look further than impact on the research process, to consider the impact of service user involvement on research outputs and wider changes in policy and practice. As other factors come into play it becomes increasingly difficult to disentangle the impact of service user involvement from other factors such as organisational research context (Minogue et al. 2005). As a result, some researchers have suggested a shift in language, preferring to focus on 'influence' of service user involvement rather than impact (Carden 2005).

Research in the UK aimed to increase knowledge of the evidence of the impact of public involvement on health and social care research. The project involved carrying out a structured review of the literature obtained from a collection of articles held by the organisation INVOLVE (www.invo.org.uk), a systematic search of electronic databases and requests for literature sent out through INVOLVE's networks. Relevant articles were identified by applying inclusion and exclusion criteria. A total of 89 articles met all the criteria for inclusion and were considered relevant for an in-depth review. This was carried out using a framework which helped with categorising the evidence of different types of impact and drawing out common themes. The review found that public involvement in research has had a variety of impacts. These are summarised below:

- *Impact on the research agenda*: including involvement in identifying topics for research, shaping the research agenda, initiating research projects, influencing funding decisions
- *Impact on research design and delivery*: including involvement in project design, research tools, research methods, recruitment, data collection, analysis of data, writing up, dissemination
- *Impact on research ethics*: including involvement in improving the consent process or improving the ethical acceptability of research
- *Impact on the public involved*: for example, attaining new knowledge and skills, and benefiting personally through a general increase in their self-confidence and self-esteem or gaining peer support and friendship, an opportunity to earn money
- *Impact on researchers*: for example, acquiring greater understanding of a health condition, or of a particular local area or culture
- *Impact on research participants*: for example, improvements to the way research is carried out by involving peer interviewers or user researchers
- *Impact on the wider community*: including creating trust and acceptance of the research, keeping projects grounded and focused on benefits for the community, improving relationships between the community and professionals
- *Impact on community organisations*: for example, staff and/or members of community organisations gaining knowledge, raising their profile, making links with other community members and making a positive contribution to the research
- *Impact on implementation and change*: such as informing the development of new services or improving existing ones, changing professional practice, establishing long-term partnerships with capacity to take action

The review also identified factors that influence the impact of involvement. The evidence suggests that public involvement has had the greatest impact when people have been involved throughout an entire research project, rather than just at isolated points. Over a longer-term, involvement is reported to have more impact because members of the public gain more insight into research, members of the public and researchers develop more constructive, ongoing dialogue and a general ethos of learning from each other is established. Other facilitating factors are training and support for the people involved and linking involvement to decision-making. The authors of the review conclude that there is a demand for more robust and rigorous methods in the assessment of the impact of service user involvement. It is also clear that much can be learnt from the powerful 'stories of involvement' told by service users and researchers. A notable methodological challenge lies in finding methods for capturing these stories in a consistent and rigorous way.

Economic perspectives of service user involvement in research are relatively unexplored, beyond issues about service user payments (see Chapter 3). Yet competition, efficiency and productivity in health care and research are increasingly important throughout the Western world. Questions about economic impact arise in relation to every area of research expenditure. Healthcare reform is being driven by attempts to fund and deliver services in a way that meets ever-increasing demands in the face of cost containment pressures. An economic analysis of service user involvement in research might look at cost against effectiveness. It may also be feasible to undertake an economic analysis of direct comparisons of alternative service user approaches, for example looking at costs of consultation versus collaboration. Economic perspectives could also be useful for informing resource allocation for service user involvement in the research commissioning process and for supporting investment in user-led research (Beresford 2003). However, health research is often commissioned through numerous separate programmes, which limits the capacity for resources to shift in response to evidence on cost-effectiveness of service user involvement.

Reporting impact

As with other types of research, it is important that research is reported clearly, with summaries available for different stakeholder groups. It is helpful to make reports navigable so that readers can 'dip in' to impact reports without having to read the whole document. Written reports should be supplemented with presentations to interested groups. Opportunities for discussion and dialogue can be critical to the dissemination process.

Web 2.0 technologies offer opportunities to share research with potential audiences in different formats and to engage with potential readers in a variety of ways. The term Web 2.0 is associated with web applications that facilitate participatory information sharing, user-centred design and collaboration on the World Wide Web. Users enter dialogue as creators of user-generated content in a virtual community, in comparison with traditional websites where users can only view content. Examples of Web 2.0 include social networking sites, blogs and video sharing sites.

Given the limited number of impact studies of service user involvement that are to be found in the published literature, a key part of any dissemination strategy should be an effort to place the results in the public domain, preferably in a journal so that it will remain accessible over time. The INVOLVE review (Staley 2009) concluded that it would be helpful to have guidelines for researchers publishing impact studies to improve consistency and allow others to judge the quality of the studies. There is a tendency to publish only positive results, yet there is scope to learn from service user involvement that has not

---

Key information it can be useful to report on:

Aims: What is the relationship between what is being assessed and research, policy and practice. What types of priorities, purposes and perspectives informed the aims and process?
Objectives: What were the main steps in carrying out the assessment? How was the assessment divided into tasks and activities?
Focus: What was the focus of the assessment? Did it include the whole research timescale and everyone involved or only certain aspects? What information was recorded?
Types of impact: What types of impact were recorded and why? (positive and negative). What was not recorded?
Timescales: How long did the research project/programme last? What was the timescale of the impact assessment? e.g. was the assessment going on during the research, after the research, or for a time during the research

---

Figure 10.4   Reporting impact studies – aims and context.

Key information it can be useful to report on:

Who was involved: Who was involved in undertaking the assessment? Who was observed/studied as part of the assessment? Why?
Methods that were used: What type of approach was used (qualitative/quantitative, mixed-method) and why? What techniques were employed, e.g. interviews, focus groups, questionnaires, documentary sources. Was a monitoring system used?
Findings: What does the study show overall? What is the degree of certainty?
Discussion: How do the findings relate to other studies and existing evidence? What needs to be done next? What are the implications of what has been found? What are the main limitations (what could you not do or what were the weaknesses)?
Conclusions: Overall, what does the study show?
Authorship: Who contributed to writing the report/paper about the impact assessment?
Acknowledgements: Who should be thanked for helping support the impact assessment?

Figure 10.5   Reporting impact studies – method and outcomes.

worked or has faced significant barriers. Writing up these experiences for publication would be beneficial for sharing learning.

It could be helpful to consider some common types of information that might be included when reporting impact (summarised by Figures 10.4 and 10.5). To guide the reporting process it can also be helpful to develop a dissemination strategy detailing planned activities and outputs.

One of the main difficulties in reporting impact is how to deal with challenging findings. For example, if the impact study finds no impact, or negative impacts, at great cost, how will this information be received by key stakeholders and those that have devoted time and energy to the research? It is helpful to consider this issue at the start of the process of an assessment. It is also a strong argument for engaging stakeholders, including service users, in the impact assessment process; to ensure that findings do not come as an unwelcome surprise at the end of the process. That said, it can be useful to have this type of evidence for developing and supporting service user involvement in future research and in reporting back to funders and stakeholders about how best to invest future resources.

Key principles for practice

- When embarking on an assessment of impact, be sure to clarify the purpose from the outset.
- Articulate your understanding of the relationship between service user involvement and research, policy and practice.
- Consider engaging stakeholders in the impact assessment process from the start.
- Consider the diverse methods available and adopt an approach that is both rigorous and likely to engage with stakeholder audiences.
- Develop a dissemination strategy and report (both positive and negative) findings widely.

References

Barber, R., Boote, J., Parry, G., Cooper, C., Yeeles, P., and Cook, S. (2011) Can the impact of public involvement on research be evaluated? A mixed methods study. *Health Expectations* (first published online 17 Feb 2011).

Baxter, L., Thorne, L., and Mitchell, A. (2001) Small voices big noises. Lay involvement in health research: lessons from other fields. (Produced by Folk.us) (Available from: htpp://www.invo.org.uk)

Beresford, P. (2003) User involvement in health research: exploring the challenges. *Nursing Times Research*, 8 (1): 36–46.

Boaz, A., Fitzpatrick, S., and Shaw, B. (2009) Assessing the impact of research on policy: a literature review. *Science and Public Policy*, 36 (4): 255–70.

Boote, J., Telford, R., and Cooper, C. (2002) Consumer involvement in health research: a review and research agenda. *Health Policy*, 61 (2): 213–36.

Boote, J., Baird, W., and Beecroft, C. (2010) Public involvement at the design stage of primary health research: a narrative review of case examples. *Health Policy*, 95: 10–23.

Carden, F. (2005) Making the most of research: the influence of IDRC-supported research on policy processes, Paper for the International conference '*African Economic Research Institutions and Policy Development: Opportunities and Challenges*', Dakar, 28–29 January 2005. (Available from: http://www.idrc.ca/uploads/user-S/11085518871Making_the_Most_of_Research.pdf)

Connell, J. and Kubisch, A. (1998) Applying a theory of change approach to the evaluation of comprehensive community initiatives: progress, prospects and problems. In: Fullbright-Anderson, K., Kubisch, A.C., and Connell, J.P. (eds) *New Approaches to Evaluating Comprehensive Community*

Initiatives: Volume 2: Theory, Measurement, and Analysis. Washington, DC: Aspen Institute, 17pp. (Available from: http://www.aspenroundtable.org/vol2/index.htm)

Cooksey, D. (2006) *A Review of UK Health Research Funding.* London: The Stationery Office.

Entwistle, V., Renfrew, M., Yearley, S., Forrester, J., and Lamont, T. (1998) Lay perspectives: advantages for health research. *British Medical Journal*, 316: 463–6.

Hanney, S., Buxton, M., Green, C., Coulson, D., and Raftery, J. (2007) An assessment of the impact of the NHS Health Technology Assessment Programme. *Health Technology Assessment*, 11 (53): 1–200.

INVOLVE (2007) *The Impact of Public Involvement on Research. A Discussion Paper from the INVOLVE Evidence, Knowledge and Learning Working Group.* Eastleigh: INVOLVE. pp. 1–4. (Available from www.invo.org.uk)

Minogue, V., Boness, J., Brown, M., and Girdlestone, J. (2005) The impact of service user involvement in research. *International Journal of Health Care Quality Assurance*, 18: 103–12.

Nutley, S., Walter, I., and Davies, H. (2007) *Using Evidence: How Research Can Inform Public Services.* Bristol: The Policy Press.

Peddie, V., Porter, M., Van Teijlingen, E., and Bhattacharya, S. (2006) Research as a therapeutic experience? An investigation of women's participation in research on ending IVF treatment. *Human Fertility*, 9 (4): 231–8.

Psillidis, L., Flach, J., and Padberg, R. (1997) Participants strengthen clinical trial research: the vital role of participant advisors in the Breast Cancer Prevention Trial. *Journal of Women's Health*, 6 (2): 227–32.

Smith, E., Ross, F., Donovan, S., Manthorpe, J., Brearley, S., Sitzia, J., and Beresford, P. (2008) Service user involvement in nursing, midwifery and health visiting research: a review of evidence and practice. *International Journal of Nursing Studies*, 45 (2): 298–315.

Staley, K. (2009) *Exploring Impact: Public Involvement in NHS, Public Health and Social Care Research.* Eastleigh: INVOLVE.

Staniszewska, S., Herron-Marx, S., and Carole, M. (2008) Measuring the impact of patient and public involvement: the need for an evidence base. *International Journal of Quality in Health Care*, 20 (6): 373–4.

Staniszewska, S. (2009) Patient and public involvement in health services and health research: a brief overview of evidence, policy and activity. *Journal of Research in Nursing*, July 14: 295–8.

UK Evaluation Forum (2006) Medical research: assessing the benefits to society. A report by the UK Evaluation Forum, supported by the Academy of Medical Sciences, Medical Research Council and Wellcome Trust, May 2006.

Chapter 11

International perspectives

Key summary points

- *Europe*: The importance of patient and public involvement in the governance of human services such as health care is widely accepted throughout the European Union. Changes have been made to legal and regulatory frameworks across the EU to support the development of healthcare services through the involvement of citizens and stakeholders in governance processes. Public understanding, support and involvement in research are thought to be prerequisites for a solid scientific base for innovation and growth.
- *The USA*: In the USA, service user involvement in research is more likely to be described as 'public participation'. Public participation is based on the belief that those who are affected by a decision have a right to be involved in the decision-making process. Public participation involves the use of techniques such as public meetings and hearings, advisory committees, interactive workshops, interviews, questionnaires, focus groups, and other methods to identify public concerns and preferences and address them during decision-making.
- *Canada*: In Canada, service user involvement is more often described as 'patient' or 'citizen' engagement' with an emphasis on involving the consumers of health services in 'patient-centred' decision-making processes.
- *Australia and New Zealand*: In Australia and New Zealand, service user involvement is more recognisable as consumer participation, and the term 'consumer' tends to be used in health policy rather than 'service user'. As with other countries internationally, in Australia and New Zealand there is a growing commitment at all levels – from consumers and community members, to health services and state government – that consumer participation is an ethical and democratic right.
- *Developing countries*: Challenges to health in developing countries are many. Developing countries need to be able to set their own health research priorities and create environments conducive to research investments. Research and innovation can in itself also be a source of socio-economic progress and economic advancement. Externally sponsored research also provides the opportunity to assist developing countries to strengthen expertise in conducting and reviewing research. A long history of community participation projects in developing countries has helped to inform more recent steps towards patient and public involvement in health care internationally, in terms of the approaches that are used to engage community members and methods of consultation.

Handbook of Service User Involvement in Nursing and Healthcare Research, First Edition.
Elizabeth Morrow, Annette Boaz, Sally Brearley and Fiona Ross.
© 2012 Elizabeth Morrow, Annette Boaz, Sally Brearley and Fiona Ross.
Published 2012 by Blackwell Publishing Ltd.

Europe

Governments across Europe face similar challenges in delivering higher levels of technically intensive health care to a growing population. The importance of patient and public involvement in the governance of human services such as health care is widely accepted throughout the European Union (EU) as being central to delivering services that meet public needs. At the same time there is increasing recognition of the potential role of third sector bodies, including voluntary and not-for-profit organisations, in helping find solutions to problems of organisation and delivery of health and social care services.

Quality of health care is a common issue of concern and policy attention for governments and other stakeholders across the EU. Changes have been made to legal and regulatory frameworks across the EU to support the development of healthcare services through the involvement of citizens and stakeholders in governance processes BEPA (2010). One intention is to make healthcare organisations and professionals more accountable to patients individually and collectively. At a patient level many healthcare organisations are now offering more opportunities for patient involvement. Greater 'transparency' in the evaluation of medicines, publicly accessible trial registers and public involvement in trial design has helped to improve public understanding of health research. For many EU countries priorities for healthcare research now include improving the quality of research reporting to professional and public audiences, and translating research findings into workable solutions for healthcare practice.

Across Europe public understanding of science, support and involvement in research are thought to be prerequisites for a solid scientific base for innovation and growth (Michael 2002). Links have been made across Europe to support capacity building and strengthen scientific expertise. Member states agreed in March 2000 at Lisbon on a strategy to make the EU the 'world's most competitive and dynamic knowledge-based economy, capable of sustainable economic growth with more and better jobs and greater social cohesion'. The EU's commitment to health research has translated into the allocation of over €6 billion to this area under the Seventh Framework Programme (FP7) for research and technological development, established for the period 2007–2013. This represents a significant contribution to European science and technology for the prevention, diagnosis, treatment and control of disease. It is designed to boost the capacity for innovation of health research in Europe. This investment will support a range of research activities and initiatives during FP7, with a particular focus on health biotechnology, translational research and the optimisation of healthcare delivery to citizens, as well as supporting EU policy needs.

Key sources for further information about developments across Europe include:

- *European Commission Research and Innovation* (ECRI) – The ECRI website is designed to help different types of people find out about European research. Whether you are a researcher or a teacher, in business or in politics, the site provides accessible information about the latest political decisions, and the latest advances in research funded by the European Commission. There is a set of online leaflets about *European*

Research in Action, written for the non-specialist and available in multiple languages. The *Guide to Successful Communications* presents an extensive bibliography about communicating scientific information and research findings to the public.

- *Europa and CORDIS* – This website is part of the European Commission's *Europa* portal where you can find out about all the aspects of EU policy and activities. *CORDIS* (Community Research and Development Information Service) is a website that is run separately and is intended primarily for current and potential participants in the Research Framework Programmes.
- *HealthCompetence.eu* – This is an interactive online platform that includes over 3,000 research projects on life science and health supported by the European Commission since 2004. It provides access to information on these research activities and results and facilitates the identification of potential collaboration partners and the setting up of partnerships between academia and industry in health research.
- The *EQUATOR* Network is an international initiative that seeks to improve reliability and value of medical research literature by promoting transparent and accurate reporting of research studies. The EQUATOR Network is an umbrella organisation that brings together researchers, medical journal editors, peer reviewers, developers of reporting guidelines, research funding bodies and other collaborators with mutual interest in improving the quality of research publications and of research itself. The aim is to develop into a global organisation covering all areas of health research and all nations, and actively involving all key stakeholders.
- *European Patients' Forum (EPF)* is a non-profit, independent organisation and umbrella representative body for patient organisations throughout Europe. Representing the EU patient community, EPF members advocate for patient-centred equitable health care, and the accessibility and quality of that health care in Europe. The *Value+* project was launched in 2008 with the aim of exchanging information, experiences and good practices among key stakeholders in relation to meaningful patient involvement in EU-funded health-related projects at both EU and national levels. Value+ produced a number of key resources: a toolkit for patients and patient organisations providing information on how to become involved as equal partners in EU-funded health-related projects; a handbook for project leaders and coordinators providing specific information on how to involve patient organisations in EU-supported project; a set of policy recommendations for policymakers on effective strategies for involving patient organisations in EU-supported programmes and projects. In addition to these three key tools, Value+ produced a database containing the results of the research on EU-supported health projects and the organisations that implemented them, developed a model for meaningful patient involvement in health care and a directory of patients' organisations in EU member states. These tools and resources can support cooperation with patient organisations in developing a project proposal, implementing a project and evaluating it.
- *The Guidelines International Network* (G-I-N) is a Scottish-based global network, founded in 2002. It has grown to comprise 93 organisations and 77 individual members representing 45 countries from all continents. G-I-N seeks to improve the quality of health care by promoting systematic development of clinical practice guidelines and their application into practice, through supporting international collaboration. The main objective of the *G-I-N PUBLIC* is to support effective patient

and public involvement in the development and implementation of clinical practice guidelines. G-I-N PUBLIC offers a forum for exchange between patient and public organisations, guideline developers and researchers.

The USA

In the USA, service user involvement in research is more likely to be described as public participation. Public participation is based on the belief that those who are affected by a decision have a right to be involved in the decision-making process. It is the general term for diverse formal processes by which public concerns, needs and values are incorporated in decision-making processes (IAPP 2007). Public participation involves the use of techniques such as public meetings and hearings, advisory committees, interactive workshops, interviews, questionnaires, focus groups, and other methods to identify public concerns and preferences and address them during decision-making. It tends to be thought of as two-way communication and collaborative problem-solving process with the goal of achieving better and more acceptable decisions.

Most recent US federal laws authorising or establishing federal programmes, including the latest health and environmental laws, contain requirements that government agencies consult with the public during the design and implementation of a programme. If money is awarded to a state, then these public participation requirements are also passed on to the state authorities. In relation to health care, research on managed care organisations in the USA has shown that patient involvement is pursued more than public involvement (Dixon et al. 2004) with the aim of giving individual patients greater say in their care and treatment choices.

The history of public participation in the USA has been influential throughout the Western world. It began in the 1930s when the size of the US federal government grew very rapidly. Government became involved in making many decisions that affected people's lives and it became necessary to delegate many of these to technical experts. Over time, many people began to feel that bureaucrats were making decisions which controlled their lives without any consideration of their views. In the 1960s, the civil rights movement challenged the presumed social consensus. On a nightly basis the public witnessed images on television of African-Americans being brutalised by the police during non-violent marches, church bombings and other racially motivated violence. The existing system of segregation was no longer acceptable. Riots in Watts, a low-income area in Los Angeles, and the riots that spread throughout major cities following the assassination of the Rev. Martin Luther King Jr., caused many government officials to question how the country was being run.

The controversy over the Vietnam War also challenged basic beliefs about America and how political decisions were being made. The ensuing Watergate scandal during President Richard M. Nixon's first term, and other revelations concerning political corruption and dishonesty, further engendered public mistrust of government. In an attempt to counteract public disquiet, Congress passed a series of laws designed to provide greater openness in governmental decision-making as well as dialogue with the public before decisions are made. In addition, many agencies have issued policies and regulations concerning public participation that reinforce requirements for public participation. Public participation has now developed sufficiently in the USA that it has become a professional specialty and many agencies require their planners and decision-makers to attend public participation training.

Key sources for further information about developments across the USA include the following:

- The Director's *Council of Public Representatives* (COPR) is a federal advisory committee made up of members of the public, who advise the National Institutes of Health (NIH) Director on issues related to public participation in NIH activities, outreach efforts and other matters of public interest. NIH selects new COPR members every year, to serve an average of four-year terms. The COPR is made up of 21 people from across the country, chosen to represent the public through an open nomination process. They are patients, family members of patients, healthcare professionals, scientists, health and science communicators, and educators. The COPR meets two times a year on the NIH campus in Bethesda, Maryland. COPR Members also participate in NIH initiatives and take part in public outreach activities throughout the year. A *Community Engagement Framework* was produced by COPR through a culmination of meetings with experts in research grant administration training, peer review, ethics, and community research and a literature review of published and non-published articles. The framework emphasises that community engagement is a process that requires power sharing, maintenance of equity, and flexibility in pursuing goals, methods and time frames to fit the priorities, needs and capacities within the cultural context of communities.
- The *International Association for Public Participation* (IAP2) was established in 1992. Some of members define themselves as public participation practitioners, and provide these services on a full-time basis within agencies, or as consultants. Many of IAP2's members, however, are planners, engineers or programme managers who see public participation as an important tool for being effective in those professions.
- The *International Association of Clinical Research Nurses* (IACRN) is a US-based professional nursing organisation dedicated to supporting educational and professional needs of clinical research nurses. The goals of IACRN focus on building quality education, training and practice in the specialty area of clinical research nursing. The goals of IACRN include promoting safety, self-advocacy and trust through community engagement in research.

Canada

Canada's publicly funded healthcare system includes ten provincial and three territorial health insurance plans. Known to Canadians as 'Medicare', the system provides access to universal, comprehensive coverage for medically necessary hospital and physician services. In this context, service user involvement is more often described as 'patient' or 'citizen engagement' with an emphasis on involving the recipients of health services in decision-making processes.

The Canadian Institutes of Health Research (CIHR) is the Government of Canada's agency responsible for funding health research in Canada. CIHR consists of 13 virtual institutes, which support a broad spectrum of health research. In 2010, CIHR sought advice on patient-oriented research in order to develop a country-wide strategy. CIHR collected input nationally and internationally from its partners at universities, hospitals, health charities, health professional associations, industry, and in the federal, provincial and territorial government. The overarching goal of the CIHR Strategy on Patient-Oriented Research (SPOR) is to translate research results into improved health outcomes for Canadians. CIHR has adopted the term *citizen engagement* to reflect the capacity of citizens to discuss and generate options independently. The term 'citizen' includes interested representatives from the general public, consumers of health services, patients, caregivers, advocates, and representatives from affected community and voluntary health organisations. CIHR is moving forward in realising a more systematic, ongoing integration of citizens' input in research priority setting, governance, and funding programmes and tools. In 2008, CIHR's Partnerships and Citizen Engagement Branch led to the development of a Framework for Citizen Engagement. The Framework identifies strategic areas of focus for citizen engagement at CIHR including participation in governance and review processes.

Key sources for further information about developments across Canada include the following:

- *Canadian Health Services Research Foundation* (CHSRF) is an independent, not-for-profit organisation with a mandate to promote the use of evidence to strengthen the delivery of health services in Canada. Current work on *Values-Based Decision-making and Public Engagement* aims to support the identification, investigation and sharing of promising practices for values-based decision-making, and explore the value of using deliberative processes. This involves asking questions such as: What models and approaches for public engagement have been adopted in Canada? How do we measure successful public engagement? How can citizens be supported in order to make informed choices about the use of health services?
- *The Patient Engagement Initiative* is overseen by the Canadian Health Services Research Foundation to financially support intervention projects that engage patients in the design, delivery and evaluation of health services, with the goal of improving the quality of care. Funded projects are encouraged to undertake an evaluation of the intervention's patient engagement processes, outputs and outcomes, including its impact on the quality of patient-centred care services. Previous studies have examined: patient engagement in a range of hospital in-patient settings, engagement of cancer survivors in improving cancer services, parent-to-parent support in rehabilitation services, as well as involving patients in developing safety indicators, and early intervention services.

Australia and New Zealand

In Australia and New Zealand, service user involvement is more recognisable as consumer participation, and the term 'consumer' tends to be used in health policy rather than 'service user'. As with other countries internationally, in Australia and New Zealand there is a growing commitment at all levels – from consumers and community members, to health services and state government – that consumer participation is an ethical and democratic right. There are clear policies and standards in place on consumer, carer and community participation in health services, as well as organisations working to promote participation in health research at a state level.

The Consumers Health Forum of Australia and the National Health and Medical Research Council worked in partnership with consumers and researchers to develop the Statement on Consumer and Community Participation in Health and Medical Research (CHF and NHMRC 2001). Consumers and researchers were invited to respond to a consultation paper and participated in roundtable discussions during development of the statement. The statement on participation was developed in recognition of the contribution that consumers can make to research, as well as their right to participate in research. The statement on participation is intended as a guide to consumer and community participation at all levels and across all types of health and medical research. It includes objectives and checklists as a starting point in facilitating involvement, including deciding what to research, deciding how to research, carrying out the research, letting people know the results and knowing what to research next.

During 2008–2009 a nation-wide survey of research-funding organisations and organisations that conduct research was performed in Australia (Saunders and Girgis 2010). Organisations were asked about consumer involvement in a range of areas drawn from the international literature. The most frequently reported involvement across both groups were: input into organisational governance, such as membership on strategic research planning or other high-level committees such as the Board of Directors; fund-raising for research; and assisting with the communication and dissemination of information about individual or organisation-wide research activities. More research funders (57%) than research organisations (40%) involved consumers in fund-raising for research and disseminating information about research. Across both groups, consumers were least likely to be involved in research policy development, research data collection and research grant review. Overall, research funders were more likely to currently involve consumers in research processes and structures. They were also over eight times more likely than organisations conducting research to involve consumers in identifying research needs and prioritising research topics; whilst organisations conducting research were more than twice as likely to involve consumers in recruiting research participants. Across both groups, practical and time constraints were reported as key challenges to involving consumers whilst guidelines on consumer involvement and evidence of effect were the most important potential enablers. More than a third of research organisations indicated that when consumer involvement was a condition of research funding, it was an important facilitator of involvement.

Several international organisations for consumer participation are based in Australia and New Zealand. Key sources for further information include the following:

- *The Health Issues Centre* is an independent, not-for-profit organisation that began in 1985 to promote equity and consumer perspectives in the Australian health system. Their mission is to improve the health outcomes for Australians, especially those who are disadvantaged. The focus of Health Issues Centre's work is mainly in Victoria but they take a national approach where appropriate to undertake: policy analysis and advocacy from consumer and equity perspectives, consumer-focused research, promotion of consumer participation, and dissemination of information.

- *The Cochrane Consumers and Communication Review Group* (CCCRG) is part of the Centre for Health Communication and Participation at the Australian Institute for Primary Care and Ageing. The CCCRG is an international collaboration of health service researchers, who as members of the Group, participate in the Cochrane Collaboration. The mission of the Cochrane Collaboration is to help people make well-informed decisions about health care. One of the main ways it plans to achieve this is by ensuring that high-quality and up-to-date systematic reviews of the effects of health interventions are made widely available. Systematic reviews are undertaken by review groups with editorial bases situated in many different countries worldwide. Each of the 52 review groups in the Cochrane Collaboration has its own scope to identify its area of study. The scope of the *CCCRG* is to undertake systematic reviews of research on the effects of interventions (particularly those which focus on information and communication) which affect consumers' interactions with healthcare professionals, services and researchers. The interventions may relate, for example, to individual use of healthcare services, or to consumer participation in health planning, policy and research.
- *International Association of Public Participation* (IAP2) is an international association of members (Executive Director based in Australia), who seek to promote and improve the practice of public participation in relation to individuals, governments, institutions and other entities that affect the public interest in nations throughout the world. IAP2 was founded in 1990. The initial mission was to promote the values and best practices associated with involving the public in government and industry decisions which affect their lives. The organisation has grown to over 1,000 members from 26 countries. IAP2 hold conferences and have undertaken work on the values and ethics of public participation.
- The *International Collaborative Indigenous Health Research Partnership* (ICIHRP) aims to address the inequalities in health outcomes which exist for indigenous peoples in New Zealand, Canada and Australia. One of the core outcomes of the agreement is to enable information sharing in the international research community concerning community ownership, engagement and involvement in research. Outcomes also include enabling direct links between researchers and organisations for the development of collaborative programmes, international exchange programmes, enabling links, skills development and information sharing, facilitating the development of strategic research priorities in indigenous health and international participation in peer review process.

Developing countries

Challenges to health in developing countries are many. The World Health Organization (WHO) estimates 14 million people die each year from infectious diseases, many of which are preventable or treatable, such as acute respiratory infections, diarrhoeal diseases, malaria and tuberculosis. Up to 45% of deaths in Africa and South-East Asia are thought to be due to an infectious disease (WHO 2000). The majority of research funding is directed towards HIV/AIDS, tuberculosis and, more recently, malaria. These conditions are of course very important but developing countries need to be able to set their own health research priorities and create environments conducive to research investments.

Research and innovation can in itself be a source of socioeconomic progress and economic advancement. Externally sponsored research also provides the opportunity to assist developing countries to strengthen expertise in conducting and reviewing research. Countries including South Africa, Brazil and India have made major investments in health research capability, followed more recently by other countries, including China, Thailand, Chile and Nigeria. However, many developing countries have to contend with poverty, war, endemic diseases, and a low level of investment in healthcare systems. These problems mean that research capacity building is often a low priority and even communicating the meaning or benefits of health and social care research can be difficult.

One of the greatest challenges is to conduct clinical trials and other forms of research in developing countries that will lead to health care that benefits the citizens of these countries. Rigorous ethical safeguards must be in place to prevent the exploitation of those who take part in the research. Following a number of international controversies, the Nuffield Council on Bioethics established a working party to consider the ethics of research related to health care in developing countries. The report of the working group recommends that research must be appropriately planned, taking account of the local context, and effectively reviewed on scientific and ethical grounds (NCB 2002). Four principles are put forward for anyone who is designing or conducting healthcare research in developing countries. These are:

• The duty to alleviate suffering
• The duty to show respect for persons
• The duty to be sensitive to cultural differences
• The duty not to exploit the vulnerable

Internationally there are hundreds of voluntary health organisations that work with healthcare professionals and researchers in developing countries to help carry out their humanitarian missions. Whilst the monetary value of international aid is estimated as being less than 10% of the costs of providing health care in developing countries, research and pilot programmes sponsored by agencies from the industrial nations have generated many of the best ideas for improving health. International health organisations are also a major source of expert technical advice and training for local health professionals.

Community participation projects identify local community leaders through which to engage communities and use community networks to communicate and consult with different groups of people (Molyneux et al. 2005). The idea of community participation in health first appeared in the early 1970s as it was becoming clearer that the basic health needs of developing countries could only be met through the greater involvement of local people themselves. The concept was formally articulated by the WHO in 1978 and was central to the strategy to achieve 'Health for All' by the year 2000.

Techniques and methods of community participation frequently follow a pattern that includes needs assessment, agreeing a shared vision, generating ideas and plans for action, putting plans into action, and monitoring and evaluating process and impact. The European Sustainable Development and Health Series (ESDH 2002) provides a concise guide to community participation for people working in local authorities, health authorities and other local health bodies who want to initiate or further develop community participation processes. The document reflects the diversity of community participation expertise and knowledge gained by healthcare workers and other profes-sionals working within the WHO Healthy Cities and Local Agenda 21 frameworks. As well as discussing the concept and purpose of community participation, it provides details of 15 techniques for engaging communities including: undertaking community profiles and appraisals, rapid participatory appraisal, guided visualisation, future search, citizens' juries, community participation advisory groups and community councils, and story-dialogue method.

Key sources for further information about developments internationally include the following:

- *World Health Organization* (WHO) is the directing and coordinating authority for health within the United Nations system. It is responsible for providing leadership on global health matters, shaping the health research agenda, setting norms and standards, articulating evidence-based policy options, providing technical support to countries and monitoring and assessing health trends. WHO carries out its work with the support and collaboration of many partners, including UN agencies and other international organisations, donors, civil society and the private sector. WHO uses the strategic power of evidence to encourage partners implementing programmes within countries to align their activities with best technical guidelines and practices, as well as with the priorities established by countries.
- *Healthlink Worldwide* is an international non-government organisation that works to improve the health and well-being of poor and vulnerable communities by strengthening the provision, use and impact of information. Healthlink Worldwide supports around 30 partner organisations in Africa, Asia, Latin America and the Middle East to strengthen their communication strategies. They work to address issues including how to support South–South links, and how to support increased dialogue between policymakers in the North and South. Healthlink Worldwide also works with government and non-government agencies on short- and long-term information and communication projects. The organisation offers expertise and training in various aspects of health and disability-related communication, including needs assessment and impact evaluation, project management, development of print and electronic materials, and resource centre and database development.
- *Health Exchange* is a forum for practitioners and frontline health workers to share experiences and lessons from the field. It is a quarterly on-line and print magazine designed to have a practical focus on important health topics. Health Exchange aims to help inform developing-country and international health practitioners, policymakers and researchers.
- *Wellcome Trust International Engagement Awards* support projects to strengthen the capacity of people in low- and middle-income countries to facilitate public engagement with health research. Projects are intended to stimulate dialogue about health research

and its impact on the public in a range of community and public contexts in low- and middle-income countries. Recently funded studies include: participative exhibitions about medical research in Malawi, radio-style interviews and music to disseminate research findings in rural South Africa, building research capacity amongst non-governmental organisations in India, and engaging low-income communities in biomedicine and bioethics in Brazil.

Key principles for practice

- Researchers should be aware that the language of 'service user involvement' differs internationally and is influenced by the types of terms which are used in health policy and professional language.
- Different countries tend to favour different types of concepts which may be related to service user involvement, for example patient-centred care, consumer engagement, patient participation, or patient and public involvement.
- Internationally there is a wide range of government and non-government funded organisations which provide information, funding and support for service user involvement activities. Government health departments and professional bodies are good starting points for further information.

References

BEPA (2010) Empowering People, Driving Change: Social Innovation in the European Union. Brussels: European Commission, 1–131.

CHF and NHMRC (2001) Statement on consumer and community participation in health and medical research. Consumers' Health Forum of Australia in partnership with National Health & Medical Research Council, Australia.

Dixon, J., Lewis, R., Rosen, R., Finlayson, B., and Gray, D. (2004) Can the NHS learn from US managed care organisations? *British Medical Journal*, 328: 223–5.

ESDH (2002) European Sustainable Development and Health Series (4) Community participation in local health and sustainable development. Approaches and techniques.

International Association for Public Participation (IAPP) (2007) *IAP2 Core Values.* (Available online: http://www.iap2.org/)

Michael, M. (2002) Comprehension, apprehension, prehension: heterogeneity and the public understanding of science. *Science, Technology & Human Values*, 27 (3): 357–78.

Molyneux, C., Wassenaar, D., Peshu, N., and Marsh, K. (2005) 'Even if they ask you to stand by a tree all day, you will have to do it (laughter)!': community voices on the notion and practice of informed consent for biomedical research in developing countries. *Social Science & Medicine*, 61 (2): 443–54.

NCB (2002) Nuffield Council on Bioethics. The ethics of research related to healthcare in developing countries. (Available online: http://www.nuffieldbioethics.org/)

Saunders, C. and Girgis, A. (2010) Status, challenges and facilitators of consumer involvement in Australian health and medical research. *Health Research Policy and Systems*, 8: 34.

World Health Organization (WHO) (2000) Communicable diseases. Highlights of activities in 1999 and major challenges for the future. WHO, Geneva.

Chapter 12

Conclusion

Key summary points

- *Summary conclusions*: We have looked at how service users may become involved in nursing and healthcare research and the opportunities and challenges this can sometimes bring. For those working in nursing and healthcare research it is important to think about service user involvement not only in terms of requirements of research or impact on the research, but also to think about what service users, and also researchers may gain from the process. Success comes from drawing out the uniqueness of research contexts and individual people and being able to demonstrate how it may contribute to knowledge and understanding. Success also requires valuing personal and interpersonal relationships and the things that make them work.
- *Service user involvement enhancing evidence-based practice*: Service user's involvement in all aspects of the research process has the capacity to enhance the evidence base for nursing and healthcare practice. Service user involvement helps to ensure that patients' individual knowledge and interests are used to counterbalance the weight of generalised evidence in decision-making processes. Nurses and other healthcare professionals can take into consideration service user perspectives about the types of evidence that are valued and privileged when making decisions.
- *Enriching professional education*: Service user and carer involvement is increasingly common across a range of programmes in higher education, but predominantly in health and social care subject areas. Courses may include sessions where service users, carers or parents teach or speak to students. It is also increasingly common for higher education institutions to incorporate service user involvement in their strategic development plans and curriculum development. Other areas of service user involvement can include teaching and learning, recruitment and assessment of students, development of teaching materials, staff recruitment and development, and research and scholarship.
- *Teaching service user involvement in research*: The chapters of this book could be used as an outline curriculum for a session or module on service user involvement in nursing or healthcare research. The topic suits a discursive and interactive approach to learning and example topics for discussion and essay questions are provided.
- *Developing professional roles*: New nursing and healthcare professional roles often include taking the lead in developing new health services where service user, and public, involvement is crucial to ensure these are appropriate. Healthcare professionals who are

---

Handbook of Service User Involvement in Nursing and Healthcare Research, First Edition.
Elizabeth Morrow, Annette Boaz, Sally Brearley and Fiona Ross.
© 2012 Elizabeth Morrow, Annette Boaz, Sally Brearley and Fiona Ross.
Published 2012 by Blackwell Publishing Ltd.

competent to involve service users in their everyday work are more likely to be well prepared to work in a world where patient and public involvement is a normal part of how health services are designed and run.

- *Securing service user's commitment to involvement*: Understanding service user outcomes of involvement could help to attract service users to become involved in research in the first place, keep service users engaged, and help to develop successful research partnerships between service users and professional researchers.
- *Further reading*: Readers who have found this book useful may also like to follow recommended further reading. This section provides summary details of other published books from health and social care about service user involvement.
- *Web-based resources*: There are many further resources available online. This section outlines useful websites that are freely available to researchers and service users.

Summary conclusions

In this book we have looked at how service users may become involved in nursing and healthcare research and the opportunities and challenges this can sometimes bring. To ensure that nursing and healthcare research is able to inform practice, the way we think about research, the questions we ask, and the approaches we take have to be grounded in service users, experiences. We have seen that there are multiple approaches to service user involvement, such as part of researcher-led or service-user-led research or part of a partnership approach. Much has already been learnt about service user involvement in mental health research, disability research, as well as other areas of health and social care research.

For those working in nursing and healthcare research it is important to think about service user involvement not only in terms of requirements of research or impact on the research, but also to think about what service users and researchers may gain from the process. There is no doubt that service user involvement can be a challenge but it is also an opportunity to develop new types of skills, insights and understanding.

Success comes from drawing out the uniqueness of research contexts and individual people. We need to give some thought to the types of relationships we have and how we develop them with other people, whether they are working in collaborative relationships or the more traditional researcher/participant model. Researchers need to be more open with service users and listen to their challenges, reflections, sense checking and critique. This takes time, and sometimes compassion, in the context of pressing research timescales and deadlines. We believe this can best be achieved when service users are engaged in respectful relationships, which enable reciprocity and co-production of research.

Success also requires valuing personal and interpersonal relationships and the things that make them work. Members of research teams should pay attention to the 'small things' that make people 'feel big'. That is, teams of service users and researchers working together can learn about the things that matter to one another. It could be general aspects of good practice – like ensuring payments are made on time, meetings are accessible and contributions are acknowledged. More often than not it is the more personal and less obvious details that make the difference, like calling someone by their preferred name or contacting them after a meeting to follow-up on an idea. Ultimately it is in the gift of each individual researcher and service user to find out how they can make the most of what matters to them.

There is good reason for research commissioners to continue to direct research resources towards supporting the involvement of service users, but there is also a pressing need to devise more structured and systematic approaches for reviewing and reporting on the investments that have been made. Involvement in research comprises many different processes and outcomes in different contexts. At the present time, learning is not routinely being captured or utilised for quality improvement. Fulfilling the promise of service user involvement in research requires doing more to build an evidence base and to understand the quality of processes and outcomes concerned. It is important that the research community strives to explain the positive interactions and successes that can happen when service users and researchers work together.

Service user involvement enhancing evidence-based practice

In this section we will look at how service user's involvement in all aspects of the research process has the capacity to enhance the evidence base for nursing and healthcare practice. Evidence-based practice (EBP) is an idea that most clinicians working in the Western world will be familiar with as it is a strong feature of health professional education and professional development. In nursing it means 'using the best available evidence from research, along with patient preferences and clinical experience, when making nursing decisions' (Cullum 2000). Evidence-based nursing (EBN) is the nursing variant of EBP, which itself emerged from evidence-based medicine (EBM). EBM has been defined as 'the conscientious, explicit, and judicious use of current best evidence in making decisions about the care of individual patients' (Sackett et al. 1996). Whilst the notion of 'best evidence' is often thought of as evidence generated by means of the randomised controlled trial (RCT) (Rothwell 2005), promoters of EBM have argued that it is not just about the application of research-trial-generated knowledge in the clinical arena, but also involves clinicians' judgements and patients' values (Sackett et al. 1996).

Evidence-based nursing has, to an extent, engaged in the issue of clinicians involving patients in decision-making about their treatment and care, rather than relying totally on evidence-based protocols (Sackett et al. 1996). However, some professionals, and patients, have criticised EBN for failing to sufficiently use patients' individual knowledge and interests to counterbalance the weight of generalised evidence. The argument is that service users are able to make judgements and observations based on their understanding of a health condition, treatment or issue and may have a different take on what outcomes are important, and that these valuable insights are not sufficiently considered alongside trial-generated evidence (Entwistle et al. 1998). EBP has not always taken into account the effects of interventions upon specific individuals or their personal preferences. EBP has also been criticised for ignoring the importance of processes in the implementation of health care, such as the significance of clinical leadership and change management expertise in utilising best evidence at a local level. Other criticisms are that it marginalises other forms of professional and lay knowledge, undermines the autonomy of patients and functions for the benefit of vested interests (Porter et al. 2011).

A positive paradigm of EBP would involve recognising the significance of individual service user's experiences of health and health care because it is these lived experiences that are the most direct and authentic forms of knowledge (Glasby and Beresford 2006). Furthermore, it would take into consideration service user perspectives about the types of evidence that are valued and privileged when making decisions. As we have shown through this book, service user involvement means the active involvement of service users in the design, undertaking and evaluation of research, rather than treating people simply as the subjects of research. Involving service users in the research process itself can improve the relevance of the research questions that are asked, and help to inform choices about appropriate research tools, approaches to data collection and outcome measures.

Enriching professional education

For many recently trained nurses and healthcare professionals service user involvement is a standard part of the training they receive. They may have learnt about service user involvement through research methods training or have experience of patient and public involvement in healthcare decision-making or practice development. Moves to involve service users in professional education are taking place within the wider policy agenda for increased public engagement in policy development, service planning and delivery. The involvement of service users and carers as partners in professional education is promoted by professional bodies such as the Nursing and Midwifery Council in the UK. Service user and carer involvement is evident across a range of programmes in higher education, but predominantly in health and social care subject areas.

In most higher education health and social care courses service users will have some direct involvement in delivering sessions, seminars or assisting with student assessments. A popular area for service user involvement is in communication skills training. At a masters and degree level it is becoming increasingly common for student assignments to incorporate an element of service user involvement. Courses may include sessions where service users, carers or parents teach or speak to students. This can include sessions using song, poetry and drama, or question and answer sessions.

Involving service users in training and education is not without its problems. Imbalances of power and control in favour of the professional and the institution are often evident. A literature review of service user involvement in healthcare education has identified a number of common challenges (Repper and Breeze 2006): students may give more credence to teacher-led sessions; adherence to the rules, regulations and traditions of academic institutions can be problematic for service user involvement; a desire to ensure academic balance to service user's accounts; a wish to promote the professional accountability of the lecturer. Not all teachers view service user involvement positively because they are uncertain about the benefits, ethical issue, or how it will affect their role and accountability as educators. The findings of the review indicate that to alleviate these problems there is a need to develop courses in partnership with service users; undertake further research on the impact of service user involvement and to track the development of organisational service user involvement strategies; and systems for supporting service users need to be established, including training for service users and staff.

It is becoming more common for higher education institutions that teach health professionals, to incorporate service user involvement in their strategic development plans. Departments and faculties may have invested resources in setting up service user and carer advisory groups to directly inform their work or to develop strategic plans for service user and carer involvement in the teaching programmes they deliver. Members of such advisory groups are typically service users and carers with experience of receiving healthcare, and staff with experience of involving patients, service users or carers in their work. Advisory groups can help to share knowledge, experiences and ideas of service users, academics and administrative staff about specific areas for service user and carer participation in departmental structures and academic programmes. They can also help to identify the skills and support required for service users to contribute to education programmes from the service users' perspective, such as helping service users to identify which aspects of their personal experience they are willing to share and providing support for teaching large or diverse student groups. Advisory groups can help to plan how to achieve parity of experience between classes, raise awareness of service user workloads and ensure that there is consistency in how service users are rewarded and acknowledged for their contributions.

Areas of service user involvement can include teaching and learning, recruitment and assessment of students, development of teaching materials, staff recruitment and development, and research and scholarship. Other forms of service user involvement are also beginning to emerge in educational institutions, for example service users teaching on some courses are involved in assessing students' presentations or practical skills within simulated clinical environments. Service users may contribute to auditing practice placements or be directly involved in student research studies. The involvement of service users and carers in health professional education means that students learn to see service users as individuals, and to recognise the value of patient and carer experience alongside broader evidence.

Guidance on how best to involve service users and carers in professional education is limited, beyond mental health, social work and learning disability. A good source of information is the Working Together Online Toolkit (www.serviceuser and carertoolkit. co.uk), funded by the Lifelong Learning Network and developed by a collaboration of academics and service users from Keele University, Staffordshire University, Open University and the University of Wolverhampton. The toolkit provides a flexible set of resources for people who work in universities in health, social care and social work departments who are considering or developing the engagement of service users and carers in teaching programmes and research. It provides practical advice and case examples which can be used to support these processes.

Teaching service user involvement in research

For readers who are also teachers, the chapters of this book could be used as an outline curriculum for a session or module on service user involvement in nursing or healthcare research, perhaps as part of a research methods course. The theoretical framework for approaching service user involvement in research presented in Chapter 2 ('Service users' section) could also provide a useful structure for a course outline covering context, methods, roles and outcomes of service user involvement. This framework, possibly used as a PowerPoint slide or handout, could enable students to visualise the issues and see how they are interrelated.

The topic of service user involvement in research suits a discursive and interactive approach to learning. For example, students could be encouraged to explore the language, concepts, models and issues that are associated with service user involvement in research through group discussion or debate. In this way it is likely that they will learn to question broader research issues about representation, knowledge and control for themselves. By way of example, the following topics for group discussion are drawn from the first two chapters of the book. They are most suitable for courses at degree level and above.

Example student group discussion topics

Perspectives and expectations of involvement

- Service user involvement in research means 'active' and 'direct' participation: when/ why might this not always be possible?
- Why is service user involvement in research a political issue?
- What are the major ethical issues when involving service users as active partners in research? How do these issues contrast with involving service users as subjects of the research?
- Although service user involvement can improve the quality of research studies there are also potential drawbacks: what might these be?

Principles of involvement

- Who are 'service users' and 'carers' – as individuals, groups and organisations?
- How does 'experiential knowledge' fit with EBP?
- Should service users have a right to empowerment?
- Are clinicians or researchers the best advocates for service users?

The principles for practice at the end of each chapter could also be developed into learning outcomes or topics for assignments, though these would need to be devised according to the appropriate level of learning and for different student groups. The following example essay questions are drawn from Chapters 3 and 4. They could potentially be used at degree level and above. It could also be beneficial to encourage students to consider these questions in relation to a specific research study (e.g. to critically review a published research paper), or a proposal for research, or their own student research projects.

Example student essay questions

Designing involvement

- Explain the range of contributions different types of service users may bring to a research study. Consider the contributions of people with direct experience of a health issue, people with direct experiences/opinions of health services, patient representatives, patient advocates, carers, community representatives, and national service user representatives, as well as seldom-heard groups.

- How might different types of service user involvement be employed at different stages of *designing*, *undertaking* and *evaluating* a research study?
- Discuss why different approaches to service user involvement (such as different levels of control and models) may be used within different research traditions and methods.
- In relation to a specific research study, break down steps of involvement according to key aims and objectives, clarify the actions and time required and who will be responsible.

Working relationships

- How might you approach service users to work with you on a specific research study? Consider your existing research relationships, clinical relationships, connections to local services, public advertisements, and service user organisations and community groups. Provide a clear rationale for who is being approached in relation to the purpose of the research and explain the opportunities for involvement.
- Devise a job role and outline responsibilities for service users involved in a specific research study.
- Develop an information sheet for service users who are going to be involved in a research study to outline the general principles of confidentiality, data protection and informed consent.
- Why is it important to collect feedback from service users involved in a research study? Explain the techniques you could use to gain feedback from service users.

Another aspect of professional education is learning to identify and examine ethical issues. The principles for practice at the end of each chapter could also be developed into practical examples of ethical issues. The following example ethical issues are drawn from Chapters 5 and 6. They could potentially be used as discussion points at degree level and above.

Example student ethics questions

Patients, clients and carers

- Healthcare professionals have a duty to provide care and support to patients. Is it ethically wrong or right to involve patients who are receiving health care in research?
- It is unethical to exclude people who are very sick from research. What types of safeguards and practical steps can be put in place so that they can be involved if they wish to participate?
- Patients with rare clinical conditions can have high hopes for what research might achieve. How would you explain what some of the limitations of research can be?
- Some potential barriers for service users to becoming involved are disability, age and ethnicity. What other types of barriers can prevent people from being involved in research?

- What does 'capacity to consent' mean? Is it always necessary in relation to involving service users as equal partners in research?

Involvement over the life course

- Children and young people can and should be involved in research when it is appropriate to do so: When might it not be appropriate?
- People who are sick or those who are undergoing treatment or care within a healthcare setting should not be unnecessarily burdened by research. Where else might it be better to recruit service users from?
- What is 'individualised communication' and how might you use it with a group of older people involved in a research study?

A further aspect of professional education is awareness of social inequalities and the cultural and personal barriers that some members of society face to social inclusion. The following example issues are drawn from Chapters 7 and 8. They could potentially be used as group work questions at degree level and above.

Example student group work on social inclusion

Seldom-heard groups

- What types of people might be described as 'seldom-heard'?
- Consider the individual needs of a person who is blind: What might they need to be able to join a research advisory group?
- Consider the communication preferences of the deaf and people who are hard of hearing at a research dissemination event: What might these be?
- How might you find out how best to communicate with a service user researcher who has learning disabilities?
- Black and minority ethnic (BME) groups may suffer racism, health inequalities and language barriers. Which BME groups are there in your area of work/region?

Service user-led research

- Consider how you might work with a volunteer network to plan a research study: How might you engage members' interest?
- Charitable organisations can be an accessible source of information about research for service users. Use the internet to identify the major charities working in your field/ research topic area.
- It is becoming more common for academic departments to employ service users: What are some of the benefits?

Part of teaching service user involvement is to encourage professional learning about research practice and outcomes. The following example issues are drawn from Chapters 9 and 10. They could potentially be used for student assignments at degree level and above.

Example student assignments on research practice and outcomes

Quality

- Explain what 'principles for successful involvement' are and give an example of how you would use them in a research study.
- Design an activities log to record service user involvement activities, explain what you would record and why.
- For one month keep a reflective diary on the subject 'My views and knowledge of service user involvement in research'.
- Research teams can work towards quality experiences of involvement by understanding the perspectives of those that are involved in the research. Design a set of questions for a 'feedback' questionnaire.

Impact

- Devise a plan for an assessment of impact of service user involvement in a research study on patient experiences of care. Explain which aspects of impact you will focus on.
- Draw a diagram or picture to represent the relationship between service user involvement and research, policy and practice. Provide a written explanation of the main features of the diagram.
- You have secured research funding to undertake an impact assessment of service user involvement in a research trial for cancer drugs: How might you involve service users in undertaking the assessment?
- You have just finished a research study on the nursing role in preventing childhood obesity. Develop a dissemination strategy to report both positive and negative findings to policymakers, healthcare practitioners and service users.

Developing professional roles

As well as keeping up with new knowledge and with changes in the health system and organisations they are working within, nurses and other healthcare professionals are taking up more and more different roles. Roles change as professionals expand existing roles. This often means that other staff are required to take on some aspects of a previous role, for example as registered nurses expand their role, healthcare support staff often take on elements of basic care which were previously part of the registered nurse role. Healthcare professionals may develop new roles which are designed to fit within their scope of practice, for example new clinical nurse specialist roles and emergency nurse practitioner roles. Such roles are an extension of professional practice for an individual group, although in some circumstances another professional group may feel that the role is equally appropriate for them. Completely new roles may be developed which do not fit existing professional boundaries, for example healthcare support staff who work between nursing, physiotherapy and occupational therapy. These roles can be filled by existing healthcare staff or by staff new to the health service with appropriate training and education.

New nursing and healthcare professional roles often include taking the lead in developing new health services where service user, and public, involvement is crucial to ensure these are appropriate. Healthcare professionals who are competent to involve service users in their everyday work are more likely to be well prepared to work in a world where patient and public involvement is a normal part of how health services are designed and run.

Little is known about how different researchers perceive their role in relation to involving service users in research. It is likely that a number of factors influence this, including policy/funders requirements for involving service users and the strategies and support put in place by research organisations. But perhaps the most significant determinant of a researcher's attitude towards service user involvement is whether they have personal experience of working with service users. Researchers frequently report that working with service users changes their attitude towards research and their role as a researcher. Some approaches to involvement require researchers to develop skills not traditionally perceived as part of the researcher role, for example skills of facilitation, providing training, encouragement and support to service uses, and communicating using accessible language.

Embedding patient perspectives in all areas of health and social care is a safeguard against the escalation of paternalistic and unquestioned professional practices. But rather than just helping to keep professionals working in a professional way, service user involvement can also be a source of inspiration for new forms of professionalism. For example, service user involvement in research extends professional accountability to the public beyond reporting research findings, towards a greater awareness of the need to 'translate' research on behalf of service users in terms of the language, focus and priorities of those research is intended to serve. The developing role of nurses and healthcare professionals requires them not only to understand research findings and to weigh-up different forms of evidence, but to generate new evidence in partnership with service users. As part of their professional role, nurse and healthcare researchers can learn about indicators of successful involvement, how to document service user involvement work, and how to make use of reflective techniques to build towards quality experiences of involvement and quality environments for involvement.

Securing service user's commitment to involvement

There is still much to learn about how best to secure service user's contributions in the context of different research settings, methods and approaches. Initiating communication between researchers and service users is an obvious first step in ensuring individuals and communities are involved in the work of research organisations. Service users need to be informed of why they in particular have been approached, what it is the researcher wants to learn and what is expected from them in the research. Researchers are sometimes concerned that service user representatives should not simply be those who are the most vocal, eloquent or communicative, because they wish to consider a range of service user viewpoints and experiences. These concerns can be alleviated by being explicit about who will be involved and why, for example stating in research proposals and protocols how service users will be recruited and the types of roles they will be asked to take on in the research. There are also the challenges of securing direct and active involvement of people from non-English speaking backgrounds, people with communication difficulties, people who do not identify themselves as 'service users' and other seldom-heard groups.

Payments and recognition for involvement are certainly important for securing service user commitment; however, involvement can lead to more personal types of benefits for service users who are involved, including improved therapeutic outcomes, better access to health information or social networks, and a sense of empowerment (Chapter 11). Understanding these types of outcomes could help to attract service users to become involved in research in the first place, keep service users engaged and help to develop successful research partnerships between service users and professional researchers. What is clear is that service users express diverse reasons for wanting to be involved in research and that they gain different things from being involved.

Stigma and stereotyping continue to be substantial barriers to involvement of some service users in research. Mental health service users, often more than any other service user group, have been assumed to be incapable of voicing valid opinion and of being unaware of their own needs and hence excluded from participating in research. In bringing together researchers and service users it is important that these stereotypes and presumptions are acknowledged, addressed and dispelled from the research. There is also a need for awareness of service user's cultural environments, including race, country of origin, and religious belief. In order for service users to be involved on their own terms, these aspects of who they are need to be understood, respected and worked with.

The relative deficit of accounts in the literature of involvement on a national scale points towards a difficulty for researchers to connect with patients and the public beyond organisational or regional boundaries. Problems are most likely to be attributable to the practical issues of scaling-up involvement and the intensive nature of participative approaches. For example, issues such as having limited time or resources, but also because of a lack of certainty about when to engage service users at a national or a local level. One solution to problems of scale is to use highly structured consultative methods, patient surveys for example, yet these have received criticism for being too prescriptive about the questions they ask and for failing to involve service users in a direct or active way in the research process.

The internet provides a powerful new tool for participation, although all its potential uses are still being discovered. In the near future, research organisations will not only use the internet to provide information to the public, but will make greater use of it as a tool for gathering public input and information. There is considerable concern, however, about a 'digital divide', as the number of people with access to the internet in some cultural groups, and the poor in general, is considerably lower than in the public at large. People fear that the increased use of the internet for research purposes will mean that minorities and the poor will not have the same access to decision-making processes as those people who are connected digitally. Consumer groups and voluntary networks, on the other hand, have embraced the internet enthusiastically, and use it extensively for organising and communication with other groups.

The internet, together with other web-based technologies, provides a new forum for knowledge creation. 'Social learning' is a new paradigm of finding, consuming, creating and contributing information via collaborative commons. In a social learning environment, online communities create and maintain multiple forms of information bases. Members of such a community are able to then find and utilise information via informal sharing. Social learning is not limited to content that has been created by the community, but it also extends to the ability to make contact with experts or build consensus of meaning about topics and ideas. Social learning can attain a high degree of engagement among participants and could offer a method of generating and spreading knowledge as one component of service user involvement in nursing and healthcare research.

For those service users who become involved in the work of established research institutions, their experiences are likely to determine whether they choose to continue to be involved. The discrepancy in the amount of power service users have in research is often made most obvious by the language used to describe their involvement, for example 'giving' service users a role in the research or 'allowing' service users to sit on research advisory groups. This language, although describing progressive ideas, can be off-putting or derogatory for service users who are expecting to be treated as equal partners. The uncertainty and complexity of research can also be difficult to comprehend and researchers need to be ready to explore areas of conceptual uncertainty with service users. For example, service users should be clear about why they are being asked to be involved in any particular research endeavour. To successfully communicate the aims or purpose of involvement researchers should be explicit about working towards a shared sense of purpose, whilst acknowledging the impact of the context within which the process is taking place. Research teams can help to contribute to securing service user's contributions by addressing the following questions:

Example questions for research teams

- Are we following principles for successful involvement?
- Are we sufficiently documenting the roles of service users in the research (e.g. maintaining an activities log about service user involvement)?
- Are we maintaining financial records of funding and payments?
- Are we reporting and acknowledging service user contributions in research reports and papers?
- Have we met service user's training needs?
- Have we sought service user's advice about recruitment and participant information?
- Are we disseminating research findings to service users and relevant service user groups in appropriate formats and easily understandable language?
- What reflective techniques are we using to examine issues about the quality of involvement processes (e.g. reflective diaries, feedback and evaluation forms or reflective interviewing)?
- Are we giving sufficient attention to the personal, interpersonal, contextual, political and ethical factors which influence the research? Are we aware of the strengths and limitations of what has been done and are we able to explain the decisions that have shaped the research?
- Do we understand the perspectives of those service users that are involved in the research, in terms of their personal experience of the process?
- How can we build more supportive research environments for service user involvement and challenge any barriers to involvement?

It is also important for research teams to include service user outcomes when recording and reporting on impact (Chapter 10). This information could help to encourage service users to become, or remain, involved in research.

Further reading

The following list contains a selection of recommended books on service user involvement in health and social care research.

- *Critical Perspectives on User Involvement* edited by Marian Barnes and Phil Cotterell (Hardcover – 1 November 2011) (The Policy Press). This book draws on contributions from user activists and academic researchers, to provide a critical reflection on the state of service user involvement across health and social care. It considers different contexts in which such involvement is taking place and includes diverse and sometimes conflicting perspectives on the issues involved. In three parts, the book looks at the rise of user movements, service user involvement in health and social care services, and service user involvement in research. It discusses contemporary issues about measuring and evaluation of public involvement in research.
- *Handbook of Service User Involvement in Mental Health Research* (World Psychiatric Association) by Jan Wallcraft, Beate Schrank and Michaela Amering (Hardcover – 17 April 2009) (Wiley-Blackwell). This book describes the relevant background and principles underlying the concept of service user involvement in mental health research, providing relevant practical advice on how to engage with service users and how to build and maintain research collaboration on a professional level. It highlights common practical problems in service user involvement, based on experience from various countries with different social policies and suggests ways to avoid pitfalls and common difficulties.
- *Involving Service Users in Health and Social Care Research* edited by Lesley Lowes and Ian Hulatt (Paperback 2005) (Routledge). This book draws together over 40 contributors from consumer groups, families and parents, and professionals from social care, healthcare and research areas. The content of the book is as mixed as the authors, from personal reflections, discussions on ethics, ideas for changes, to descriptions of actually fulfilled projects and their impact. It covers a broad range of issues on the theme of professional and service user partnerships.
- *User Involvement and Participation in Social Care: Research Informing Practice* by Hazel Kemshall, Rosemary ed. Littlechild, and Rosemary Littlechild (Paperback – 7 July 2000) (Jessica Kingsley Publishers). This book is written by researchers and practitioners working in evaluation research. It is concerned with key themes: research methodologies which promote 'just' inquiry, research methodologies which mirror goals of participation and involvement, commitment to mutuality, ways in which service users can be engaged in research, techniques for involving respondents about the findings of research, involvement of service users in decisions about the outcome of the research, and the role of participants in evaluating the research process. The authors draw upon empirically based studies in the areas of health, social care and criminal justice.

- *Service User and Carer Involvement: Beyond Good Intentions* by Mo McPhail (Policy and Practice in Health and Social Care Series) (Paperback – 29 November 2007) (Dunedin Academic Press). The authors of this book are a service user consultant, a carer consultant and academics from three universities in Scotland. They write about their individual and collective experiences to communicate learning about service user and carer involvement at local, institutional and nation levels in the fields of health and social care and in professional education. Chapters focus on themes including intentions, power, voice, expert knowledge, ways of knowing, frustrations and possibilities.
- *Service User Involvement: Reaching the Hard to Reach in Supported Housing* by Helen Brafield and Terry Eckersley (Paperback – 15 December 2007) (Jessica Kingsley Publishers). Drawing on original research, this book offers imaginative and effective strategies for consulting with service users who have been historically hard to reach, including homeless people, care leavers, ex-offenders, travellers, women escaping domestic violence, and black and minority ethnic groups.
- *This is Survivor Research* edited by Angela Sweeney, Peter Beresford, Alison Faulkner, Mary Nettle and Diana Rose (2009). Ross-on-Wye: PCCS BOOKS Ltd. This book gives clear explanations of the terminology and theory of research. It is a useful and relevant tool for both service users and professionals involved or simply interested in survivor research. The book covers a wide range of issues facing service users/survivor research in the climate of social inclusion such as the meaning of objectivity, validity and reliability when engaging as a service user in research.

Web-based resources

There are a growing number of resources available online; some well-established sites are listed below.

- Healthtalkonline (www.healthtalkonline.org)
  Healthtalkonline is the award-winning website of the DIPEx charity. DIPEx has created two websites – www.healthtalkonline.org and www.youthhealthtalk.org – of people's experiences of almost 50 different illnesses and health conditions. The websites are aimed patients, their carers, family and friends, doctors, nurses and other health professionals and are based on in-depth qualitative research carried out by the DIPEx Health Experiences Research Group at the University of Oxford.
- INVOLVE (www.invo.org.uk)
  INVOLVE is a national advisory group, funded by the National Institute for Health Research (NIHR). Its role is to support and promote active public involvement in NHS, public health and social care research. INVOLVE publications include guides for researchers, members of the public and research funders. INVOLVE produces a newsletter and holds conferences every two years. *Putting it into Practice* is a new database on the INVOLVE website. It provides useful information on good practice, reports of the lessons learnt from direct experience of involvement, and descriptions of involvement in research projects. The database can be found on the resources area of the INVOLVE website. INVOLVE have produced a *Public Information Pack* for members

of the public who are interested in getting involved in health or social care research. The pack is made up of four booklets which cover the kinds of information people need, when first getting involved in research as well as a 'jargon buster' providing a glossary of some of the words used in research.

- InvoNET (www.invo.org.uk/invonet)
  InvoNET is a network of people working to build evidence, knowledge and learning about public involvement in NHS, public health and social care research.
- National Institute for Health Research – Research Design Services
  In the UK, the National Institute for Health Research (NIHR) has established a network of Research Design Service (RDS) to help researchers develop and design high-quality research proposals for submission to national, peer-reviewed funding competitions for applied health or social care research. NIHR Research Design Services all provide web-based support and resources for patient and public involvement in research.
- NHS Evidence – Patient and Public Involvement (www.library.nhs.uk/PPI)
  This website contains collections of clinical and non-clinical resources within specialty themes. The PPI specialist collection aims to support the implementation of patient, user, carer and public involvement in health care by providing access to the best currently available information which is freely available on the web.
- People in Research (www.peopleinresearch.org)
  This web-based resource is aimed at members of the public in the UK who are looking for opportunities to get involved in research activities. Researchers and research organisations can advertise their opportunities on the website and you can sign up to receive email alerts on a chosen topic or activity.

References

Cullum, N. (2000) Users' guides to the nursing literature: an introduction. *Evidence Based Nursing*, 3 (3): 71–2.

Entwistle, V., Renfrew, M., Yearley, S., Forrester, J., and Lamont, T. (1998) Lay perspectives: advantages for health research. *British Medical Journal*, 316: 463–6.

Glasby, J. and Beresford, P. (2006) Who knows best? Evidence-based practice and the service user contribution. *Critical Social Policy*, 26 (1): 268–84.

Porter, S., O'Halloran, P., and Morrow, E. (2011) Bringing Values Back into Evidence-Based Nursing: The Role of Patients in Resisting Empiricism. *Advances in Nursing Science*, 34 (2): 106–118.

Repper, J. and Breeze, J. (2006) User and carer involvement in the training and education of health professionals: a review of the literature. *International Journal of Nursing Studies*, 44 (3): 511–9.

Rothwell, P.M. (2005) External validity of randomized controlled trials: to whom do the benefits apply? *Lancet*, 365: 82–93.

Sackett, D., Rosenburg, W., Muir Gray, J.A., Haynes, R.B., and Richardson, S.W. (1996) Evidence-based medicine: what it is and what it isn't. *British Medical Journal*, 312: 71–2.

Index

Note: Entries shown in *italics* denote figures.

Handbook of Service User Involvement in Nursing and Healthcare Research, First Edition.
Elizabeth Morrow, Annette Boaz, Sally Brearley and Fiona Ross.
© 2012 Elizabeth Morrow, Annette Boaz, Sally Brearley and Fiona Ross.
Published 2012 by Blackwell Publishing Ltd.